Ask
DR. ANNE

Anne Hogsett, MD

Order this book online at www.trafford.com
or email orders@trafford.com

Most Trafford titles are also available at major online book retailers.

Print information available on the last page.

ISBN: 978-1-4907-9104-3 (sc)
ISBN: 978-1-4907-9103-6 (hc)

Library of Congress Control Number: 2018959087

Trafford rev. 10/05/2018

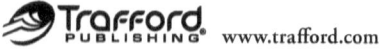 www.trafford.com

North America & international
toll-free: 1 888 232 4444 (USA & Canada)
fax: 812 355 4082

Introduction

Dr. Anne Hogsett is the Director of Hospital Medicine at Coffeyville Regional Medical Center in Coffeyville, Kansas. In March of 2016, Josh Umholtz, the publisher of the newspapers in both Coffeyville and Independence, Kansas (The Coffeyville Journal and The Independence Daily Reporter) asked Dr. Anne to make a volunteer contribution to the health of the region by writing a weekly column in which she would answer any questions submitted by the newspapers' readers. The column ran for 53 weeks in 2016 and part of 2017. So many people were asking for copies of previous columns that Dr. Anne decided to put all 53 columns in book form.

Dr. Anne would like to remind everyone that as we continue to study, our understanding of medicine will change AND medical recommendations will change accordingly.

Now that this book is finished, Dr. Anne is hoping to get started again. So, if you have more questions, send them in and then pick up the following week's newspaper to get your answers!

Chapter 1

HOW TO FEEL BETTER

Dear Dr. Anne, I'm one of those people that never feels good anymore. So, I'm ready to get healthy – where do I start? Signed R. from Independence

The absolute most important thing that you can do for your health is to realize that the little decisions you make every day, not can have, but DO have a huge impact on your health over time.

God made our bodies so that we can recover from so many things. The problem is when we continue to do things that are bad for us; eventually our bodies can no longer recover. For example, we all know that smoking is the most common cause of emphysema and chronic bronchitis (lung disease). But, if you stop smoking soon after you start, then studies show that you are much less likely to have chronic lung disease when you get older.

Or say you overindulge on alcohol on Saturday night. Many of us have made that mistake, so you know it will not kill you. But if you overindulge on alcohol EVERY Saturday night, there is no doubt that your liver will be damaged and eventually you will have liver disease.

I had a patient who had a sensitive stomach and she found that a peppermint candy seemed to soothe her stomach. So she started eating peppermint candies constantly throughout the day to keep her stomach settled. So, yes her stomach didn't hurt as much, but she was bathing her system in sugar all day, every day and after a few years she was diabetic.

If you decide not to exercise for a week while you are on vacation, your body can recover when you start exercising again. But, if you decide that your only exercise will be the time you spend walking around Walmart, then your muscles are going to atrophy (which means the muscle cells die and are not replaced) and you will have many, many further complications.

In reality, there's no such thing as one disease process. That means that if you have smoked enough to have lung disease, you will also have heart disease and peripheral vascular disease. If you have liver disease, it's going to cause heart and kidney disease. If you're diabetic, you are going to end up with heart disease, and most probably kidney disease, vascular disease and neurological disease.

The key to a life of good health is making good decisions every day, or at least as often as you can. If every day you decide to smoke one less cigarette, or eat an apple instead of a cookie, or increase your walk time by even two minutes, the cumulative effect of those changes will be huge. It is the little decisions, made every day, that make the big differences in your health.

Chapter 2

LOW BACK PAIN

Dear Dr. Anne, what can I do about my low back pain? Signed D. from Independence

Great question and since so many of us suffer from back pain, this is a very relevant question. First, you need to know that about 50% of the population has degenerative joint disease of the spine by the time we are 50 years old, which means that the pain will come and go with changes in weather, exercise level, certain foods that your body may find inflammatory, and stress level.

Before we go any further, EVERYONE needs to know the warning signs of nerve damage. So, if you have new onset loss of bowel or bladder control when you are having an acute episode of back pain, then you are most likely going to need surgery and you need to be seen by your doctor. In the same way, if you have new numbness or weakness in a leg during an episode of low back pain, then you need to be seen by your doctor.

Now that we have the scary stuff taken care of, it is back to the basics and in the case of back pain, the basics are key. So, first and foremost, you must keep the muscles of your back in shape. The great news is that the exercise required to keep your back in shape takes minutes a day. Here is an easy way - everyday lie on

3

your stomach on the floor and arch your back while you lift your arms and legs, count to 10 and then relax, and repeat. Increase the time you spend arching your back as you are able. This will take, literally 2 to 5 minutes a day, but it will make all the difference in the world. Also, get on line and Google "low back stretches," then pick five and do them at least 5 days a week. You will need to do your back exercises and back stretches regularly for the rest of your life - or as long as you would like to avoid back pain.

This second basic is harder to do, but equally important. If you are 100 pounds overweight, your low back is just going to hurt. Nothing can prevent that. Our bodies were not designed to handle that kind of weight. So do whatever it takes to reduce the weight and your back pain will decrease.

Basic point three is that you need to see a chiropractor regularly. Even if your weight is perfect, your muscles can pull your vertebrae out of alignment. If you have a time of higher stress, or you strain your back moving something heavy, or even if you step outside in 20 degree weather and the muscles of your neck and back tense in the cold wind, the muscles can actually pull the vertebra out of alignment. If that happens it puts pressure on a nerve and you will have pain! Now, if you don't like being twisted or wrenched around, just tell them. There are other ways for the chiropractor to adjust you.

But, even if you do all of those things, there are still going to be low back pain exacerbations. It just happens, so when it does you can take the following over the counter medications:

Acetaminophen – buy 500 mg tablets and take up to 3,000 mg in a 24 hour period. I usually say two tablets, three times a day. Unless you choose to drink alcohol that day, then you need to decrease your dose, because your liver is going to have to choose which to break down and it will choose the Acetaminophen leaving the alcohol as a toxic metabolite.

If that is not enough, AT THE SAME TIME, you can take:

Naproxen Sodium – 220 mg tablets, and take up to 3 tablets twice daily with food. The only people who can't take this one are those with heart failure, kidney failure, or ulcers.

(Some people don't feel that Naproxen works for them, but Ibuprofen does. For those people, instead of adding Naproxen to the Acetaminophen you can add Ibuprofen. Take 800 mg of Ibuprofen up to three times daily with food.)

If that it still not enough, go see your primary care provider and ask for a very short course of steroids – although, I have to admit that the efficacy of steroids are controversial in this case and your provider may not be willing. There are also prescription muscle relaxants, but I have not found them as beneficial as we all hope. And, my personal favorite – MASSAGE! I love that treatment option, and it is justified. Studies actually show that it does help – yeah!

Studies also show that you should NOT stay in bed! Crazy right? But, studies show that getting up and walking as much as possible will help resolve the exacerbation faster.

Most importantly, you must know that exacerbations of back pain usually last 6 WEEKS. In most cases, nothing is going to make the pain go away immediately. But, if none of what I have listed above helps, then it is time to see a surgeon, and amazingly we have one here in Montgomery County, Dr. G. Hsu and I can confidently assure you that he is an excellent surgeon.

Chapter 3

SPIDER VEINS

Dear Dr. Anne, here is a photo of one of my ankles. My skin didn't used to look like this, so what is going on? Signed V. from Independence

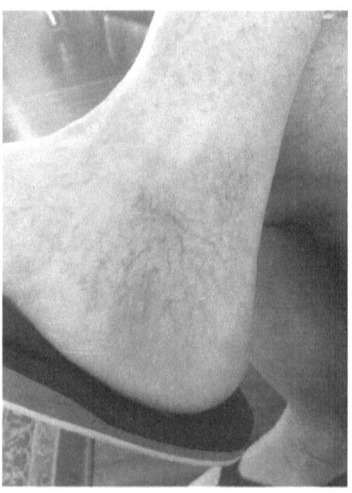

Dear V., Those are referred to as spider veins. They are similar to varicose veins, but much smaller and they are part of the natural wear and tear on the body, darn it. It is caused by the weakening of the walls of our tiny superficial veins.

Are they preventable? No, not really. Things that MAY help are regular exercise, keeping your weight within the normal range, wearing support hose when you are going to have to stand a lot, putting your feet up when you can relax, and wearing flat heeled shoes which increase the work of your calves. But, I can tell you that I have patients who do, and have done, all those things, and they still have spider veins.

The good news is that they are treatable. There are several ways to treat them, but the best way that I know of is with an injection of a chemical called a sclerosant, that is known to cause inflammation to those tiny veins. This basically kills those tiny vessels so that blood no longer flows through them and they no longer show. There are several different sclerosants that are used, but you don't need to worry about that, it is up to the doctor.

So, how does the treatment work? You make an appointment with an office that offers spider vein treatment; they will likely require a consultation appointment first and then you have a follow up appointment for the procedure. (Usually the cost of the consultation visit will be deducted from the cost of the treatment, but you will need to count on the treatment costing about $350-$450 and, of course, this is cosmetic only, so your insurance will NOT help with the cost.) The needle used for the treatment will be tiny, not only very short, but also not very big around. You will lie on the table and they will inject a tiny amount of sclerosant into each area that you want treated, up to a certain amount of sclerosant in a single visit. There will be some stinging, but really not much.

The hard part comes after the procedure, because you will be required to wear prescription compression pantyhose, usually with 30-40 mmHg compression. You will need to wear them for 24 hours a day for 3 days after the treatment (which means you will put them on as soon as the treatment is finished). You will wear them all day and all night for the first 72 hours. Then you will need to wear them only during the day, but will be allowed to take them off at night, for several weeks after that – depending on the doctor's instructions, but usually 3 weeks.

As many of us know, prescription compression stockings are VERY hard to put on AND they are HOT. So don't do this in the summer. You have to be measured for prescription panty hose and they cost between $130 and $200, which is a lot. But, you have to have them tight on your ankles and/or calves - wherever the sclerosant has been used. You also need to know that you will not have complete resolution for about 3-4 months AND, of course, you can get more spider veins at anytime because they are part of aging. So, you may have to repeat the process.

It is one of those decisions that we women fight all the time; how much am I willing to do? Dye my hair, or not; perm my hair, or not; wear make-up, or not; fight the continual onslaught of facial hair, or have my friends call me Jeff.

Chapter 4

METHAMPHETAMINE

Dear Dr. Anne, I want to know what is so bad about meth? I have lots of friends that use meth and they are just fine. AND, I know adults who have been using meth for years and they are just fine, so what is the big deal? Signed C. from Independence

Dear C., I am so glad that you asked me about methamphetamines, or meth. Unfortunately, meth has very serious long term effects.

Let's start with the effects on the teeth. I am sure you have heard of "meth mouth." Unfortunately, this can develop very quickly, in some people just months after regular use of meth. In other people it takes a few years. There is no single reason that meth mouth happens, but it is a common and well documented problem.

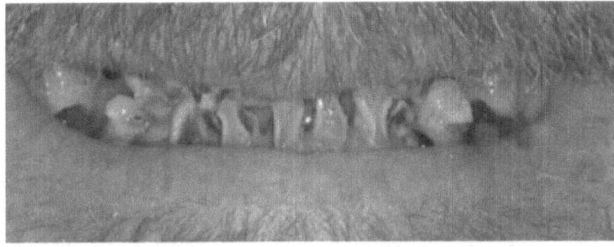

I have had patients who want to use meth, but don't want to end up with meth mouth, so they have decided to inject the meth into their veins. This is NOT a brilliant idea. When you break the skin barrier with a needle and push that needle into your vein, you are very likely to push bacteria and toxins straight into the blood stream and you can end up with bacteria growing in your blood, on your heart valves, as well as abscesses that can show up just about anywhere on the body. That black part in this photo is dead, rotting skin caused by bacteria that entered this patient's body after injecting meth.

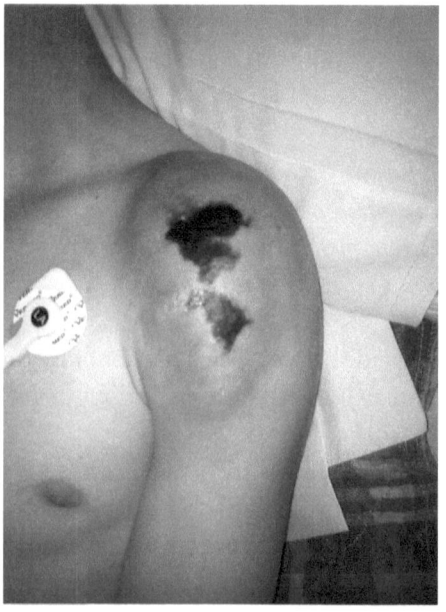

Meth use is known to cause high blood pressure, erratic heart rhythms, and over time heart failure. The heart beats in a 2-stroke system with the top of the heart squeezing first and the bottom of the heart squeezing second. Meth damages the tissue of the heart muscle, so that the electrical impulse from the top of the heart cannot travel down to the bottom of the heart. Then the squeezing of the top of the heart and the bottom of the heart are not coordinated. This is known as complete heart block, obviously a very serious life threatening situation. I have personally seen this happen, in meth users *here **in Montgomery County***.

Meth use also causes changes to the brain itself. It is known to block the dopamine receptors, which also causes Parkinson's Disease, so meth users can end up with a Parkinson's-like disease. It also causes visual and auditory hallucinations, as well as paranoia and other forms of psychosis. It causes memory loss and stunts the development of emotional maturity. Probably the biggest immediate problem is that it causes aggressive, belligerent behavior, which is why most of the arrests in our county involve someone who is using meth and hurting someone else.

C., if you know people that have been using meth for years and "are just fine," then I ask you, are these successful, happy, productive people? Are they leading lives that that you would like to lead? If so, they are the lucky few, because I am taking care of a lot of meth users with heart failure, huge skin infections and paranoid psychosis. And, those people are NOT happy people.

Many of us do stupid things when we are young. But, if we stop doing them, we at least have a chance to laugh about those stupid things and grow up. Unfortunately, meth is *extremely* addictive and there is just no such thing as "meth in moderation." Caffeine is a moderate drug, methamphetamine is not. And, I promise you, that the effects of meth on your body will not be moderate either.

Here is the really hard part. If you are surrounded by people who are meth users, the chances are very good that you will eventually end up doing the same thing. You must find someone else to be around. The truth is that we humans tend to do what those around us do. If those around us sit and eat junk all day, we tend to do the same. If those around us work and exercise daily, we are more likely to do the same. If those around us are drinkers, we tend to be drinkers. That's the way we humans are. Make your choices carefully, C. No matter how old you are, your life is important and you have great potential. Meth use will DESTROY that potential.

Chapter 5

HYPERTENSION

Dear Dr. Anne, I never had high blood pressure before, so why do I have it now, and why is it important to control my blood pressure anyway? Signed B. from Coffeyville

First, the most important reason to control your blood pressure is because long term high blood pressure (also called hypertension) is the number one cause of strokes, the second most common cause of kidney failure (which means you end up on dialysis or die), and a common cause of heart failure. Most of us cannot tell when our pressures are high and that is why hypertension is called "the silent killer."

The guidelines for blood pressure control changed in about 2013. At that point the new guidelines said that if you are under 60 years old you need to keep your pressure below 140/90. If you are over 60 years old, you need to keep your pressure below 150/90. However, it is a little more complicated then that. If you have chronic heart disease, kidney disease, chronic obstructive lung disease or diabetes, then you need to stay **below** the 130/90 mark. AND, your blood pressure should ONLY be taken when you are sitting with your legs uncrossed, with your arms at rest, and only after you have been sitting quietly for at least 5 minutes.

What causes high blood pressure? Some of the things that cause high blood pressure are "modifiable" meaning that we can change them, and some of them are not. First let's talk about those things that are NOT modifiable or just part of the aging process.

Just like our skin loses elasticity with age, the same thing happens with our arteries and the valves of our hearts. The arteries can lose their elasticity and stiffen; you've heard the term "hardening of the arteries." Well, imagine that your arteries have lost their ability to relax to accept the big surge of blood that comes from the heart with each beat. In this case, the heart is going to have to push harder to get the blood into the small opening of a tight, stiff vessel. Similarly, over time our heart valves get stiff and the heart has to push harder to get them to open. Both these factors increase the pressure that the heart has to generate to move the blood.

But, what about those modifiable causes of hypertension? A high salt diet can increase your blood pressure, if you have salt dependent hypertension. I know this is confusing at first, but if you have high blood pressure because you have stiff, calcified vessels, then salt may not make that much difference. But, there are those of us whose high blood pressure is caused and worsened by how much fluid we have on board. If that is the case, then you need to avoid salt. A logical next question would be, "How can I tell?" Well, keep track of your blood pressure, taken at different times of the day, always as I outlined above. Then increase or decrease the salt content in your diet and see if your pressure is affected. The fact is that most of us have more than one problem, so if you have high blood pressure, it is likely being caused by more than one thing and reducing your salt intake will likely help.

Alcohol consumption is another common modifiable cause of high blood pressure. Smoking can cause high blood pressure. Anything that irritates the vessels or causes plaque build-up (like diabetes, cocaine use, or eating bad fats and sugary foods, or starchy foods) can cause high blood pressure. As always, a healthy diet and regular exercise are absolutely critical in preventing and treating hypertension.

Now, you might be saying to yourself, "I don't care if I have high blood pressure. I love having my scotch every night and if I die, then I die." The only problem with that reasoning is that a stroke will likely not kill you, just leave you debilitated, or with a personality change. Not great options in my mind. But, you don't have to make changes over night. Remember, those small changes make a big impact over time. Cut back where you can, and increase exercise where you can, and watch your blood pressure control improve.

Chapter 6

CHRONIC CONSTIPATION

Dear Dr. Anne, The older I get the more I struggle with constipation. Do you have any constructive advice? Signed T, from Indendence.

Thank you for asking about chronic constipation. I really can't understand why I am completely thrilled to discuss this subject, but I am. Thank goodness I found medicine, right?

So, the vast majority of the time constipation can be managed with dietary changes, bulk-forming agents, laxatives and/or enemas, and we will discuss all that, in detail, below. But, there are a few who have a defecatory disorder, which means there is a problem on the back end. So, if we try everything else and nothing works, you may need to go to a specialist who can perform anorectal manometry (a test to see if the muscles are working appropriately) and a balloon expulsion test, which even I don't want to think about.

But, on to the run-of-the-mill chronic constipation, the first thing to realize is that not everyone has a stool every day. But, all of us should "go" at least every fourth day. Anywhere in between multiple times a day, and every 4th day, is normal.

We also need to make sure that you are not taking a med that is causing the constipation or worsening your natural tendency toward it. A quick list of medications that are notorious for causing constipation are: antihistamines, antidepressants, antipsychotics, iron supplements (sometimes calcium supplements), antacids, sucralfate, ANY opiate (tramadol, hydrocodone, oxycodone, methadone, hydromorphone, etc.), some blood pressure meds, and some chemotherapy meds. Tons of us start taking a daily antihistamine because we struggle with allergies and don't realize that it is contributing to chronic constipation. If you are not sure about your meds, ask your doctor.

There really is no substitute for drinking water when it comes to constipation. Without a doubt, drinking more water helps. Prunes and prune juice are NEVER a bad idea for those who suffer with constipation. And, colonic motility is highest in the mornings and after meals, so those are good times to drink a big glass of water and sit on the stool with something to read to see if you can "go." There is nothing wrong with sitting there a few minutes to give your body a chance to work, just don't stay there an hour – hemorrhoids anyone?

The next most important thing is bulking agents – psyllium (Metamucil or Konsyl), methylcellulose (Citrucel), polycarbophil (FiberCon), or wheat dextrin (Benefiber). These are all good for colonic health and the treatment of constipation, just try each until you find one that is the least offensive and take it daily. But, remember that they MUST be taken with plenty of water or you can just end up more plugged than before.

Then there are stool softeners, which cause the stool to absorb water and make it not so hard. Examples are docusate sodium and docusate calcium and they can also be purchased over the counter. Many patients find that these make things easier. But, there are two things that you must remember. First, stool softeners are NOT laxatives – that is, the will not stimulate your bowels to move. They just make the poo soft. And, unfortunately, in most people, they should not be used for chronic daily use. Your body will become tolerant of it and instead of 1 tablet twice daily, you will start to need more and more medication.

So, let's move on to osmotic agents. These cause intestinal water secretion and increase stool frequency. The most common is polyethylene glycol. I am sure you have heard of GoLYTELY, which is of course a lie, and MiraLAX, which is a much more reasonable drug. There are others, magnesium citrate can be chilled in the fridge and it kind of tastes like sparkling mineral water, kind of. Mag Citrate is fast acting, but also causes a lot of abdominal cramping. I would probably choose MiraLAX if you need to use something regularly and magnesium citrate for those times that you might need something extra.

I know this may feel like it is getting long, but how can you be bored? It's medicine! Next, there are the stimulants. These alter the electrolyte transport of the mucosa and increase the intestinal motor activity – that means they force your bowels to move. There are tons of these. A couple of examples are bisacodyl (Dulcolax) and senna (Senokot and Senokot-S), but any of the over the counter meds are ok to use. Just remember, that you cannot know WHEN they will make your bowels move.

Then there are enemas. In the hospital I usually start with a warm water enema. If that is not successful, then a soap suds enema, then a mineral oil enema, and if none of those work then a milk and molasses enema usually works (it is exactly what it sounds like). However, there are times that I have to bring out other things that are not available over the counter, but since we are talking about out-patient medicine, we won't discuss those. Fleets enemas are my least favorite, because they can cause problems reacting with other meds and causing allergic reactions.

There are also suppositories, the most common are glycerin suppositories or bisacodyl suppositories. Glycerin is more gentle and is often used for children, but both are effective.

If you have gotten really impacted there are times when dis-impaction is necessary. Before you attempt this, you could try a mineral oil enema to soften things up. Either way, get a pair of gloves and get it done. *IF* all of that doesn't work, go to the ER, but only if you have exhausted your options at home.

Finally, don't forget that what you eat truly does matter. The old saying, "An apple a day, keeps the doctor away" was talking about avoiding constipation! An apple won't solve current constipation, but it will keep you from getting constipated.

Now, wasn't that fun? Who doesn't love this stuff?

Chapter 7

DIET AND EXERCISE AS WE AGE

Dear Dr. Anne, I'm a male in my late 60's. I've got several questions. (1) I've read that as we age we're going to lose muscle mass. I do some modest weight lifting several times a week. Is it hopeless? Do we all turn into flab regardless of our exercise routine? (2) Do I have to eat a decent breakfast? The older I get the less I can consume on a daily basis and maintain my weight. I'd rather have a very small breakfast (like a couple of cookies), a light lunch and a reasonable supper. It seems to work. Am I inviting any problems with that system? (3) What really happened to the dinosaurs? (4) If I have beachfront property, will it wash away in the next few years? Signed, D from Independence.

Dear D from Independence, thanks for writing in. These are great questions.

First, you are absolutely right, that the vast majority of us have to eat less as we age or we will continually gain weight. There are many reasons for this – but changes in activity level and changes in hormone levels, are key. (I am not just talking about testosterone and estrogen, but hormones that regulate water balance, kidney function, bone structure, digestion, liver function, thyroid and parathyroid hormones and many more.) What is most important is that we all recognize this as being absolutely true and it is a normal part of the aging process. We simply cannot allow ourselves to eat what we ate 10 years ago and maintain the same weight.

And if you're serious about eating nothing but cookies for breakfast I will smack you silly. Cookies are edible, but have no nutritional value. You would have more energy and likely lose weight if you switched your two breakfast cookies for two breakfast eggs – cooked any way you like.

I have seen a few patients who, once they turn about 85 or so, don't seem to need to control what they eat quite so much, and they can still maintain their weight. It seems that, in these folks, the body gets a little less efficient and so they can actually increase their intake. But, I need to stress that this does not happen in everyone or even in most people.

That leads us right into your question about continuing to work out and trying to maintain muscle tone. You are again right, that we all tend to lose muscle tone as we age as it definitely gets harder to maintain or build muscle with increasing age. The natural decrease in testosterone and estrogen with aging is a huge part of this and it is inevitable. Not to be too graphic, but the real tragedy is when someone has not maintained muscle tone OR a reasonable weight. The inevitable result is that they can no longer take care of themselves, and caregivers are required to lug and lift, just to keep the individual clean. So, please, please, do not stop your modest weight lifting and exercise program. It is wonderful that you are doing it and it will save you and your loved ones much grief later on.

As to the demise of the dinosaurs, I have no idea. But, in reference to your beachfront property, I can tell you that it is pretty much worthless and you should gift it to Gary and me right away, to save yourself the heartache. Why don't you bring the deed and meet G and me for dinner Tuesday night at Uncle Jack's?

Chapter 8

CELIAC WITH HIGH CHOLESTEROL

Dear Dr. Anne, I have celiac disease and have been on a gluten free diet for years. Now my doctor tells me my cholesterol is 235 and I need to change my diet. Can you give me some suggestions for a gluten free diet that will also keep my cholesterol down? Signed E from Independence

Dear E, First, please accept my apology for putting off answering your question. I have been struggling to decide how to answer it in a newspaper column; it would be so much easier face to face.

For my other readers, who have not had to live with Celiac, it is an autoimmune disease that causes inflammation of the small intestine. Those who have Celiac are genetically predisposed to have it, then something happens to trigger or "turn on" the reaction to gluten. (There are a number of theories about what those triggers are, but we are not sure at this point.) Usually, the problem shows up in childhood, but occasionally we may not figure things out until adulthood. Diagnosis is made with a combination of blood tests and biopsies of the small intestine. The problem is that if you have been avoiding eating gluten for some time prior to the testing, you may test negative even if you actually have the disease.

The ONLY cure for celiac disease is to avoid ALL gluten. That means that you avoid ANY form of wheat, barley, rye and triticale (which is a cross between wheat and rye). That doesn't sound like all that much at first, but, it is easy to get tripped up on a gluten free diet because (1) there are other names for wheat flour, like durum flour, farina flour, graham flour, kamut, semolina (that is what pasta is made from), and spelt, and (2) so many foods have some form of gluten in them, like: beer, breads, cakes, pies, cereals, communion wafers, cookies, crackers, croutons, French fries, biscuits, gravies, imitation meat or imitation seafood, matzo, pastas, processed lunch meats, salad dressings, soy sauce, thickened soups and soup bases, etc. and (3) because even non-gluten containing grains are often contaminated with gluten in processing.

Those with Celiac really do have a tough road. So, I can see why adding concerns for cholesterol would seem overwhelming. I have good news, but again, it is not easy to explain and some would say controversial.

In the 1980's significant medical research was concluded that many researchers and doctors now feel were mis-interpreted. In the 80's we told everyone that fat in our diets was making us fat, giving us coronary artery disease and giving us colon cancer. As a nation, we cut way back on red meat, eggs, and cheeses. And, the American food manufacturers responded by filling the supermarket shelves with thousands of fat free cookies, fat free candies, fat free salad dressings, fat free sour cream, etc. Unfortunately, instead of cholesterol levels decreasing, or the incidence of coronary artery disease decreasing, or the incidence of diabetes, or hypertension decreasing, the exact opposite has happened. We now have much more obesity, much more diabetes, much more heart disease, etc.

What we now believe is that a diet high in sugar, simple carbs, and processed foods, is the real cause of elevated cholesterol.

So, V, my suggestion is to continue with your gluten free diet. If there are any simple carbs that you can cut out, do so. That is ANY form of sugar (like candy or ice cream) or starchy foods (like fries, chips, rice, sweetened nuts, etc.). If you have already done all of that, then you must increase your level of exercise.

I hope that you are not discouraged after reading this. Adding more restrictions to your diet may seem overwhelming, but frankly, cleaning up for the cholesterol is nothing compared to what you have been dealing with for years. And the exercise will release endorphins and make you feel stronger and lighter on your feet. You can do it V! Don't give up.

Chapter 9

DR. PEPPER

Dear Dr. Anne, can you please settle a disagreement. My wife and I have been married for 20 years and my wife still weighs exactly the same she did when we got married; she looks fantastic. I, on the other hand, do not weigh the same that I did 20 years ago. She fixes us three really healthy meals a day. But I also drink two Dr. Peppers each day, one lasts me all morning and the other lasts all afternoon. I drive to the Jump Start and fill up my "mega-mug" each time, which holds 44 ounces. So here's the disagreement: I say that my weight gain is genetic and is to be expected. She says that the Dr. Pepper could be responsible for my weight gain. What do you say? F from Independence

Dear F, I'm surprised to hear that you've been married for 20 years and have not yet learned the two most basic rules of being married. Here they are: Rule #1, Your wife is always right. Rule #2, If your wife is wrong, see Rule #1. The sooner you get that, the happier you'll both be.

Okay, so that was a joke. Your wife may enjoy it, although you may not.

But in total seriousness, let's do the math. Search the internet on your smart phone or computer for "Nutritional information Dr. Pepper." You'll see that Dr. Pepper has 25.6 grams of sugar for an 8 ounce serving. Even allowing some room in your mega-mug for ice, you're probably getting about 60 ounces of Dr. Pepper per day (30 ounces in the morning and 30 ounces in the afternoon). Consuming 60 ounces at 25.6 grams per 8 ounces equals 192 grams of sugar per day. There are 453.6 grams per pound, so you're consuming 0.423 pounds of sugar per day, just in your Dr. Pepper alone. You say that you do that every day, so multiplying 0.423 pounds per day by 365 days a year equals 154 pounds of sugar per year just in your Dr. Pepper (and that is conservative by allowing for a lot of ice).

At this point, please refer back to rule #1, as your wife is totally correct. Consuming 154 pounds of sugar a year is an unconscionable amount of sugar. You didn't say how much weight you've gained, but if you've been following this pattern for some time, I'm guessing that you're significantly overweight just from the Dr. Pepper. (154 pounds of sugar x 2 cups per pound x 773 calories per cup = 238,084 calories per year from your Dr. Pepper. Keep in mind that it takes 3,500 extra calories to put on a pound of fat.) I don't know how your body responds to sugar, but if I had that much extra sugar in a year, I'm 100% certain that I would outweigh the Titanic.

Please, please, please make a change right away.

My husband is also a Dr. Pepper addict. It took some time for him to wean himself off the real thing. He started out by filling his cup about a quarter full with Diet Dr. Pepper, then filled the rest with regular Dr. Pepper. After a week or so, when he acclimated to the taste of that, he filled up his cup halfway with the diet stuff, then filled up the rest with the full strength stuff. After another week or so, he graduated to ¾ diet and ¼ full strength. Then he made the leap to only Diet Dr. Pepper. The NutraSweet in the diet pop is NOT particularly healthy stuff, and I'd much rather he drink water, but sugar is an absolute killer, especially in the amounts you're now drinking.

You say that you appreciate your wife looking fantastic; I bet she'll love seeing you looking fantastic again also. I am absolutely sure that she would love for you to no longer have joint pain and low back pain, which I am certain that you have. This is not to say that people with a normal weight will not have osteoarthritis, most everyone will. But, those of us who are overweight will have a lot more daily pain.

You can do this, B. You are worth it and your wife is worth it and you are going to feel absolutely wonderful when you get all that sugar out of your system!

Chapter 10

THE PROSTATE QUESTION

Dear Dr. Anne, I am a 69 year old male, do I really have to have a prostate exam or a PSA test every year? D from Independence.

Dear D, Your question about the validity of the PSA test and the prostate exam is an excellent one, because it requires that we talk not only about prostate cancer, but also about appropriate screening for prostate cancer. So, let's talk.

About 15 years ago, the medical community recommended that ALL men over the age of 50 have a yearly prostate exam and/ or a yearly PSA (prostate specific antigen) test, which is a blood test. Then, if there was an abnormal exam, or an elevation of the PSA, we recommended a prostate biopsy. This way we caught a lot of prostate cancers early. Unfortunately, although problems are uncommon, prostate biopsies are not without complications. But, we, the doctors, felt that the benefit of finding the cancer early was worth the risk of the complications.

Then, about 7-10 years ago a very important study was published in which they studied the cadavers of several thousand elderly men, NONE of whom died of prostate cancer. And they found that a very large percentage of them had slow growing prostate cancer. Again, NONE of these men had passed away as a result of the prostate cancer that they had. We started to understand that many prostate cancers are so slow growing that they will not kill the patient. So, the question became, what is appropriate screening for prostate cancer? Are we doing a lot more prostate biopsies than we need to? And, the medical community decided that "yes," we were doing too many biopsies and we needed to back off.

In fact, the current recommendation is that the primary care doctor should sit down and discuss all this with each male patient to educate them on the pros and cons of prostate cancer screening, the prognosis of prostate cancer, the treatment of prostate cancer, the complications of treatment, and together the patient and the doctor should decide how often the patient will have a prostate exam and/or a PSA test. Unfortunately, the reality is that Medicare and insurance companies will only reimburse a doctor $63 and some change for an hour long visit, which is not enough for the doctor to pay the salaries of the employees, much less the rent on the building. So, even though the recommendation is to "discuss prostate screening with each male patient," the doctor quite simply does not have the time. Thank goodness you've got me!

So, as the patient, how should you proceed? The prostate exam is distinctly uncomfortable for most people AND if the physician does not do a lot of prostate exams, they may miss the subtleties of a small abnormality or nodule. In my opinion, the PSA (again a blood test) is a nice alternative. I think it is reasonable for men aged 50 to 80 to have a yearly, or every other year, PSA test when they have their other routine blood work. However, once a man is about 80 years old, it is not as important to check the PSA. Quite bluntly, even if there is a prostate cancer, it is unlikely that the cancer will grow fast enough to cause him a problem. However, you, at 67 should probably still have a PSA test done regularly. And, if I were a man, I wouldn't let anyone do a digital rectal exam on me unless my PSA was well into the abnormal range. But, that's just me.

Chapter 11

SUGAR ALTERNATIVES

Dear Dr. Anne, In reference to what I call your "War on Sugar," I know that too much sugar is bad, but NutraSweet is worse. So, I say it is better to drink my regular Pepsi. Signed, P from Independence

Dear P, I love your "War on Sugar" comment. I may embroider it on a pillow or better yet, have it tattooed on my bicep. Let me make my response very clear. Sugar is really bad stuff. I personally see the results of excess sugar debilitating and killing people daily. I've never seen anyone killed by NutraSweet.

So let's discuss your comment on aspartame, also known by its brand names NutraSweet, Sugar Twin, and Equal (the blue packets). I do NOT recommend these products, although the vast majority of the population does NOT have a noticeable problem with them. However, these products are known to cause neurological difficulties in people who are sensitive to them. Others can develop a sensitivity to them over time. Most often the symptoms are mild forgetfulness, confusion, or headaches. But, I have also seen patients with an increase in nerve pain. For example, these products can exacerbate (or worsen) peripheral neuropathy (pain or numbness that starts in the feet) so often seen in diabetic patients. I have also seen patients who have had rotator cuff surgery, knee or back surgery, who have increased pain after ingesting aspartame.

I even had a wonderful patient who worked really hard at her lifestyle with exercise and weight loss and did very well, but about a year later, she began to have over all, whole body pain. I did a huge work up, but could not find the source of her pain. After several weeks and many tests, she went home frustrated. Luckily, a few days later, a friend of hers recommended stopping her daily Diet Cokes and within 2-3 days her pain was resolved. I was very upset that I had not thought of the Diet Coke, but I will never forget that case.

So, NO, I do NOT recommend making aspartame part of your daily diet. (Also, remember that you cannot cook with aspartame.) Just as an aside, aspartame is made of aspartic acid and phenylalanine and is about 200 times sweeter than sugar.

However, that is not the case with all sugar alternatives. So, let's quickly review the options for sweetening your food that are NOT sugar.

Honey is a very nice alternative to sugar, because it does have some health benefits. It is known to help desensitize those with pollen allergies. **But**, it must not be given to babies and it **DOES** spike your blood sugar just like regular sugar. So, if you are diabetic or trying to lose weight, you need to avoid it.

Agave is a sweet liquid (like syrup) that comes from a plant and it doesn't crystalize like honey does. It stirs well into hot or cold and just tastes sweet, more like corn syrup. Unfortunately, it has a very high percentage of fructose, the sugar that comes from plants. It does have a lower glycemic index than glucose or sucrose, which is normally considered a good thing. (Recall that glycemic index is how much a food will increase your blood sugar.) Unfortunately, although fructose doesn't load your blood with sugar, it does load your **liver** with sugar. Which means that if you are diabetic, you liver is going to be dumping sugar periodically into the blood and you are going to struggle with your blood sugar levels. So, if you are diabetic or pre-diabetic, agave is not necessarily better than sugar.

Sucralose is a non-nutritive sugar alternative, the majority of which is not broken down by the body. That means that most of it passes right through without having any effect. You taste it on your tongue and that is about it. Sucralose has a glycemic index of zero. There have been over 110 studies completed on sucralose and most showed no significant adverse effect (one study showed that it is not good for your friendly gut flora). Although water is much better for you, there are calorie free soda pops that are sweetened with Sucralose: Sparkling ICE, and American ICE are two of them. I feel safe recommending these.

Splenda is the brand name of the sugar alternative that contains the most amount of sucralose; these are the little yellow packets. However, remember that if you actually look at the ingredients on the little yellow packet, the first ingredient is dextrose and **then** sucralose. And what is dextrose? It is a form of glucose – which is the form of sugar that has the highest glycemic index. So, you still have to be reasonable with how many little yellow packets you consume in a day.

Saccharine has been around for a long, long time. It was actually first produced in 1879 – crazy right? The brand names of saccharin containing products are Sweet N' Low, Sweet Twin, and Necta Sweet. In the 1950's and 1960's it was found that saccharin caused bladder cancer in rats, so a warning was placed on all saccharin containing products. Then, in 2000 it was found that rats have higher urine pH, higher urine calcium phosphate levels, and higher urine protein levels than humans. Apparently, in the rat bladder environment saccharin caused crystals to form in the urine which damaged the lining of the rat bladder causing the formation of tumors. As it turns out, none of that is true in human bladders. So, now the warning has been removed. But, here again, if you check the ingredients of the little pink Sweet N' Low packets, dextrose will be the first ingredient. You will not get bladder cancer, but it you eat enough of it, your blood sugar will go up.

Don't get me wrong. Both the yellow packets and pink packets are better than sugar, but moderation will be key.

Stevia is a ground leaf that is sweet. Most of the products that are sold as stevia actually are Rebiana, which is a derivative of stevia. Truvia is usually Erythritol and Rebiana. Erythritol is a sugar alcohol with a glycemic index of zero, which means that it does not increase your blood sugar at all.

But, again, you have to be savvy. At the grocery store, have you seen the big green bag that says on the front "100% Natural Stevia" next to all the other sugar alternatives? Well, if you read the ingredients list, the first one is dextrose and the second ingredient is stevia. It is still much better than sugar, but again, you will need moderation.

There is also acesulfame potassium, which we have probably all had because it is often added to packaged foods, but I cannot recall eating it on purporse.

The newest sugar alternative that I have read about is neotame, which like aspartame, is made of aspartic acid and phenylalanine. However, the chemical structure has been changed so that instead of being 200 times sweeter than sugar, like aspartame, neotame is 8,000 times sweeter than sugar – or so I have read.

Finally, there are tons of combinations and tons of sugar alcohols. I cannot cover them all, but remember that sugar alcohols are not all alike. Some have a high glycemic index others have a high glycemic load, and some are laxatives! So be careful and know what you are eating.

I know reading all this feels daunting, but you should be safe with sucralose or stevia/Rebiana. But, remember, your body is priceless. If you had a Lamborghini, would you put Mountain Dew in the gas tank? Of course not. Feed your body the best, most healthy food that you can afford. You are worth it.

Can you honestly say that ice cream is better than fresh cold watermelon on a hot summer night? Or fresh peaches in the summer time? If you want to pour some cream on those peaches go ahead. That is NOT going to hurt you, but peach ice cream or peach pie (both having been made with sugar) will.

The next time you are supposed to bring something to share, instead of cookies made with sugar, use your imagination, or the internet, and find a healthy alternative. When you find a good recipe share it! Wouldn't it be amazing if in the next census, Montgomery County, Kansas was found to the healthiest County in Kansas instead of one of the least healthy, which is where we are now? You can do this – WE CAN do this – let's do it together!

Chapter 12

OBSTRUCTIVE SLEEP APNEA

Dear Dr. Anne, the love of my life snores like a freight train. We have heard of Obstructive Sleep Apnea, should we be concerned? Signed, M from Independence.

Dear M, AND anyone who snores, AND anyone who loves someone who snores (that should be all of us). The answer is "possibly." And for now, let's just call Obstructive Sleep Apnea, "OSA."

When you go to sleep, your mind puts your body in a special housekeeping mode. During sleep, the brain works on problems that you have been trying to figure out, it tries to erase the stresses of the day, and "resets" you, so that you are ready for the new day when you wake up. In good sleep, the brain is in a calm, resting, happy mode.

When we sleep, and especially when we sleep on our backs, our lower jaw, our tongue, and other soft tissues in our oropharynx relax. When those tissues relax they can occlude (or block off) your airway, which means that you cannot get air into your lungs. If this happens, the brain says, "Uh…hey guys, we're not breathing. Everybody stop working and pay attention! We are not breathing! OMG, we're still not breathing, we're not breathing!! Is someone holding a pillow over my face?! AHHH! Wake up!!" And the brain then shoves you into the "fight or flight" mode. Your heart rate goes up, your blood pressure goes up, your blood sugar goes up, and your cortisol level goes up. That forces you to wake up enough to take a deep breath, and immediately, the brain says, "Oh. It's okay, we just took a breath, we are okay." Then you go back to sleep, only to repeat this pattern over and over again. Someone who has really severe sleep apnea will go through this cycle many, many times a night.

Sometimes people will get so revved up they can't go back to sleep at all. Others just finally wake up feeling exhausted. So, one sign of OSA is that you fall asleep during the day when you really don't mean to, during a meeting, when watching a movie, or while stopped at a stop light. Or, a patient may tell me that they wake up every night at 3 a.m. with their heart racing and they can't get back to sleep for several hours.

Untreated OSA is a really big deal and doctors take it very seriously. Over time, untreated OSA causes hypertension, weight gain (up to 12 to 13 pounds a year even with a good diet), chronically high blood sugars (which can lead to diabetes), elevated heart rate, and even atrial fibrillation (which is a huge risk factor for stroke).

So, how do we find out if someone has OSA? We do a sleep study. The best way is to go to a hospital or a sleep center where someone monitors you while you sleep and records how many times you have an "apneic event," (how many times you stop breathing). However, some of us are totally creeped out about someone watching us sleep, plus sometimes insurance won't pay for the "in house" sleep study. Luckily, there are home sleep studies, where the doctor orders the test and the company sends you a kit and instructions and then you send back the results after you spent the night being monitored at home.

When we first found out about OSA, we just told people to tape a tennis ball to the back of their sleep shirt so that they could not sleep on their backs. Then some brilliant folks came up with a CPAP machine (which stands for Continuous Positive Air Pressure) that pushes air into the airway. Some people love the CPAP from the first night that they try it, but others really struggle with feelings of claustrophobia. The masks have gotten much, much smaller and more comfortable, and the machines are now essentially silent. But, some people still struggle. Studies have shown that if someone will stick with the CPAP every night for two months, they will never give it up because they feel so much better once they get used to it.

There are also Mandibular Advancement Devices. Your mandible is your lower jaw. Basically, this is a mouthpiece that holds the lower jaw so that it cannot fall back and occlude the airway. We have dentists in the area that can make these for you and they have been shown to be just as effective as the CPAP. Unfortunately, they are not always covered by insurance. And, I must mention that these also take some getting used to and your jaw may be sore for the first 2 weeks or so. In addition, some types have an adjustable metal piece that sticks out in front and rubs on the inside of your lips causing chronic irritation and sores.

Finally, patients with OSA can also be evaluated by an Ear, Nose and Throat doctor, who may feel that it would be beneficial to remove the tonsils or any other tissue that could be contributing to the obstruction. However, these procedures are not recommended as often as they used to be. They just haven't been found to help all that much.

As an internist, I deal with chronic diseases; lung disease, heart disease, liver disease, kidney disease, etc. People generally don't get "well," we just try to help them manage their disease better. But, with OSA, once someone starts consistently wearing the CPAP, they really feel better. They are rested and energetic again. I love it when someone tells me, "I have my spouse back!" It makes my month!

Chapter 13

DEPRESSION IN THE ELDERLY

Dear Dr. Anne, I am 84 years old and my doctor thinks I am depressed. I say that I am NOT depressed, I am simply being realistic about my usefulness from here on out. Signed, H in Independence

Dear H, The easy answer is that depression in the elderly often presents much differently than it does in younger people. Instead of the usual flat expressionless face or tearfulness, elderly patients often just feel useless. It is great that your doctor is paying attention and willing to help. And, it's important to deal with this before you get so low that you are no longer getting out of bed. But, there is a broader answer that I think is much better.

I recently read a speech by Supreme Court Justice Clarence Thomas and something he said made me think of us, here in Montgomery County, and of you in particular. To paraphrase, he said that he grew up in a small farming community, and that the overriding message from his parents was that each of them had an obligation to work the land to the very best of their ability, because doing so provided for not only their family, but their community. And without optimal effort and commitment from each of them, there was no chance for independence, self-sufficiency, or freedom.

It made me think of where we find ourselves in Montgomery County today, and where you and so many of our retired folks are. It is easy to live our quiet lives taking care of only ourselves and of our own, without looking at the broader community. But, Montgomery County needs more effort than that from each of us, including YOU. Our area needs each of us, no matter how old we are, to step up and give our very best effort. We cannot afford to wait for someone else to do this for us. More importantly, YOU cannot wait for someone else to do this. You need to make the effort for your psychological health, and the area needs your effort to continue to grow and prosper.

Let me explain. You, H, have talents and knowledge that need to be passed on. If you know how to crochet or knit or embroider, what if you called one of the elementary schools and volunteered to teach your craft to a child after school? A friend of mine here in town recently showed me how to knit and it meant so much to me, but in the life of a child, it means even more.

If you are one of those lucky people blessed with a green thumb, what if you taught one child the joy of gardening? Have you noticed how few of our younger generation know how to plant and tend a garden? They have never experienced the feeling of accomplishment of picking produce or flowers that they have grown themselves.

If you are one of those rare people who can work on cars, what if you passed on your knowledge to one high schooler? Mechanical ability is irreplaceable and it gives independence, confidence, and a marketable trade.

If you are a strong swimmer, teach someone that life skill. How often do we lose someone in our local lakes or rivers because they are not strong swimmers?

If you are a rancher or a hunter or a fisherman, pass on that knowledge and those skills. These are not intuitive, they must be taught and taught carefully for safety.

In Independence, our wonderful head librarian is absolutely dying for volunteers. Please call or go by. CRMC is always looking for volunteers of almost any age. Come on down.

What if your contribution is nagging three friends into going for a walk with you every day? You know I would love that! Or maybe you are going to meet with some friends to exercise at the park every evening. Gary was in Lawrence a few months ago and commented to a resident that everyone seemed so fit. He was told that one man started exercising at the downtown park and invited anyone to join him. Apparently it has now been on going and growing for years. There are routinely over 100 people that join him to exercise!

If those are not your thing, be a surrogate grandparent. There are so many parents who are struggling. Take a kid to church, or just be there for support and guidance.

Find a charity that you want to support with your time, or your effort, or your funds. Give it everything you've got H. None of us know when our time is up, but statistically, you need to get on the ball.

There is no doubt that it will, at times, be frustrating, but I bet in the 84 years of your life, you have already been through much tougher times than what you will see with extra volunteering. Feelings of uselessness or worthlessness are cardinal signs of depression. But, I guarantee that you are NOT useless. Your wisdom and experience are needed and giving to others is a huge part of treating depression. Please don't give up on yourself; the rest of us have certainly not given up on you.

Chapter 14

SALT OR NO SALT?

Dear Dr. Anne, can you please address SALT? I love it and I need to know if I should avoid it. Signed L, Independence

Dear L, the whole salt question is a very interesting one, which as you know, means that I would love to talk about it.

Salt is actually NOT harmful for most people. In fact, the ONLY people who need to control their salt intake are those with hypertension (high blood pressure), heart failure, or kidney disease. If you don't have any of those, you don't need to worry about salt intake.

That being said, even if you don't have any of those three conditions, you may notice that when you eat a lot of salt, you feel tight or a little puffy afterwards or the next day. That is a natural reaction and over the next four days or so, your kidneys will get rid of the additional water that the salt made your body hold on to. The salt has not hurt your health, but if you don't like that feeling, I would avoid a heavy dose of salt in the future.

What if you do have hypertension? Not all hypertension is salt driven, but it is common enough that you will likely want to curtail your salt intake. One good way to find out is to eat a heavy dose of something salty and then check your blood pressure over the next 48 to 72 hours. If you notice that you are higher than normal, then you know that you are salt dependent and you need to cut back.

If you have heart failure, you need to dramatically control your salt intake. It usually does not matter what type of heart failure you have; salt in your diet will cause you to hold onto fluid, which will over load your heart and make your heart failure worse.

Many patients hope that they can eat what they want to and then increase their diuretics ("water pills") to pull the fluid off afterward. But, that only works for a while and it depends on the health of your kidneys. The bottom line is, if you have heart failure, you need a low sodium diet. That means NOT just avoiding the salt shaker, but also avoiding ANYTHING that is high in salt – like chips, almost any canned vegetable (unless it says low salt, or low sodium), sausage, bacon, beef jerky, almost any canned soup, the list goes on and on. I know it is a pain in the backside, but you are going to have to read the nutritional labels on the back of the package and keep track of how much sodium you are taking in.

If you have kidney disease and you are already on dialysis, they will dialyze off the extra salt every time you go in. But, if you have kidney disease and are not yet on dialysis, or are approaching dialysis, a high salt diet will certainly put you on dialysis faster. Dialysis will save your life, but it is not an easy way to live. For someone with chronic kidney disease, a low salt diet is a must.

I imagine that your next question is, "How much salt is okay?" The answer is, of course, it depends on your condition, and how your body reacts. This has to be discussed with your doctor. It may be enough to hold your intake to under 2300 mg of sodium a day, which is a pain, but not so bad. But, it may need to be held as low as 1500 mg per day, which is much more difficult, but still doable and worth it.

Of course, the best thing to do is to start exercising every day and eat ONLY nutritious foods. That way you will minimize your chances of having any of the problems above and if you already have one of those, you will get the most out your life in spite of your organ damage.

This is NOT easy, I know, because I love salty foods, but you can do this. No matter what the condition, daily exercise and avoiding junk food will help your heart, your kidneys, and your blood pressure.

Chapter 15

WHY SO MUCH CERVICAL CANCER?

Dear Montgomery County, I have loved getting your questions and addressing them and I look forward to continuing to do so. But, now I have a question for you. Why am I seeing so many cases of cervical cancer? Signed, Dr. Anne Hogsett

Let me explain. From all of the current medical research, cervical cancer is caused by one thing and one thing only and that is HPV (Human Papillomavirus Infection). This is a sexually transmitted disease that can be asymptomatic (meaning there may be no symptoms whatsoever), or it can cause warts anywhere on the body, or it can cause changes in the cellular structure of the cervix that leads to cervical cancer. It all depends on the strain of the virus. This is NOT to say that those with cervical cancer have been promiscuous. Remember, as far as sexually transmitted diseases go, if you have sex with one person without a condom, then you have essentially just had sex with everyone who has ever had sex with that person, and everyone who has ever had sex with those people! So please, please use a condom and protect yourself.

But, that is just background. My question to Montgomery County is... Why am I seeing so many cases of cervical cancer?

Those changes in the cellular structure of the cervix, which I mentioned above, can be detected very early by a pap smear. If caught early, it can be dealt with very easily and there is absolutely no reason for that individual to have ANY further disease process.

We have three very talented Ob/Gyn doctors (Dr. Miller, Dr. Gibson, and Dr. Lin) right here in our county and they all do pap smears. We also have a number of other doctors, nurse practitioners and physician's assistants, many of whom also do pap smears. And, FREE pap smears are offered every year through CRMC.

Let me be completely clear. Cervical cancer is completely preventable with regular pap smears! It is breaking my heart to see so much cervical cancer in our area. Advanced cervical cancer is not something you want. If I could choose the way that I will die, cervical cancer would NOT be my choice.

Earlier I said please, please wear condoms, and I meant it. But, I am also saying, please, please, PLEASE get regular pap smears! It is crazy not to. Just do it! Let's change this trend right now! No more cervical cancer in Montgomery County! Get your pap smears and let's be free of this dreaded disease.

Chapter 16

WHO NEEDS PAP SMEARS?

Dr. Anne, last week you talked about cervical cancer. I am 62 years old, and have had a hysterectomy. My primary care provider is telling me that I still need pap smears every 5 years. My question is why? From R in Independence

Dear R, your question is fabulous and I would ask the same! But, let's get into a little more detail.

First let's clarify a couple of terms. A vaginal exam examines only the vaginal canal. A pap smear gathers cells from the cervix to test for abnormalities. The cervix is the area at the opening of the uterus, which is at the back of the vagina.

So, who needs pap smears? The committees who review all the data and decide who needs pap smears currently agree that anyone who is sexually active between the ages of 21 and 65 needs regular pap smears. The definition of "regular" keeps changing, but right now that is every third year as long as there are no irregularities. If there are irregularities, then they will need to increase the frequency of the exams to monitor changes. And, remember that the definition of "regular" will likely change again.

You may ask, why not earlier than age 21 if that person is sexually active? The answer is that regardless of sexual activity, we get a lot of insignificant abnormalities prior to age 21. Remember that when we are screening for disease – in this case for cervical cancer, we are trying to find a system that catches as much of the disease as possible without causing adverse side effects. Before age 21, the pap smear can show irregular cells, but so far, they have never been shown to lead to cervical cancer.

I should have said this last week, but please vaccinate your children for HPV. There is no reason to hesitate, just do it.

You may also ask, what about other sexually transmitted diseases? Do they need vaginal exams? And the answer is, "Yes," if the patient is sexually active, and if there are problems like discharge, rash, warts, pain, ulcers, burning, itching, new unilateral joint pain without a history of trauma, or large lymph nodes.

You may further ask, why no pap smears after age 65? Well, as I said last week, cervical cancer is caused by the HPV virus and that is a sexually transmitted disease. Many people over the age of 65 are no longer at risk for exposure to a sexually transmitted disease. Either they have been in a steady relationship for many years, or they are not interested in a new relationship, or have no opportunity for a new relationship. But, let's be clear! If you are over 65, you still have a cervix, AND you have a new or multiple sexual partners, you are at risk for cervical cancer and you need pap smears. It doesn't matter whether Medicare or your insurance company will pay for it or not. We have had cases of cervical cancer over the age of 90 in our area.

You said that you have had a hysterectomy. If you had your hysterectomy because of abnormal cervical cells or a diagnosis of cervical cancer, then even though you no longer have a cervix, you still need pap smears. The doctor will just scrape the area that used to lead to your uterus to make sure that there are no abnormal cells.

If you had a hysterectomy for endometriosis, or heavy bleeding (which is called menorrhagia), or fibroid tumors, then you NEVER have to have a pap smear again!

Continuing with your question, do you need a vaginal exam without the pap? Well, are you having problems like burning or itching, pain with intercourse, bleeding after menopause, or discharge from the vagina? All of these may require a vaginal exam without a pap smear. If you are not having any problems you should not need a vaginal exam ever again.

There are only 2 exceptions to all this. First, if your hysterectomy (which means a surgical removal of your uterus) for some reason did not include the removal of your cervix. Clearly, if you have a cervix you are back to square one with regular pap smears between ages 21 and 65. The second exception is that if you had a hysterectomy, but not an oophorectomy (that is the surgical removal of your ovaries). If you had your hysterectomy early (by that I mean prior to the usual age of menopause – if you had your uterus removed in your 30's or 40's) then they usually leave the ovaries so that you can still make estrogen. If you have ovaries, but no cervix or uterus, you still need to have a bi-manual exam of those ovaries. A bi-manual exam is when the doctor puts 2 fingers in the vaginal canal and then uses the other hand to feel the ovaries for abnormalities. These are most important between the ages of 50 and 65 or if you are having problems of any kind.

I love that your primary care provider is being very careful and it drives us all crazy when the recommendations keep changing. But, right now, if you have no cervix, and your hysterectomy was not due to a cancer or abnormal cells, your insurance will not cover a pap smear, because it is not recommended. I hope that I have covered it all, but if there are other questions, please send them on.

Chapter 17

DON'T GET LAZY ON THE BASICS

Dear Dr. Anne, I am a 76 year old female in good health. The only prescription I take is for hypothyroidism. What are the most important things I need to do to remain independent and productive if I should live to be 100? Signed N, from Coffeyville

Dear N, First, congratulations on being so healthy. For a fit individual like you, we just have to concentrate on the basics.

First, stay mobile. Walk every day, and I don't mean walk around the grocery store. Walking every day for exercise is critical if you really want to remain viable. If your only walking takes place at the grocery store, it doesn't really count because you take a few steps, then stop to look at an item. This type of walking does not work your heart, or even your legs for that matter. Initially, walk as much as you're able, but try to work up to 30 minutes a day.

Second, we've got to follow a healthy eating plan. My idea of a healthy eating plan may be different from what others have told you. Concentrate on eating meats, eggs, vegetables, fruits, and dairy without added sugar. Regardless of your weight, sweets are never healthy. Even if someone is underweight, feeding them sweets to gain weight is never a good idea. Newest research shows that even those with a healthy weight, but poor muscle mass have a high mortality rate. Daily exercise and maintaining healthy muscle mass are critical.

Third, after age 65, we've got to keep in mind that we must work to prevent osteoporosis (weakness of the bones that can lead to fractures). So, getting enough calcium and Vitamin D every day is essential. Further, you need to add some modest weight bearing exercises. While twenty minutes, 2 times a week on a weight machine, or carrying 2-pound hand weights as you walk are great options, lifting your grandkids or your dog is good too. If you are not a walker, try being a dancer! Definitely, be a hugger. The more active you are, the more active you will stay.

Other things that have been shown to increase longevity are actively volunteering, having close personal relationships, having pets, and challenging your brain by learning new things. How about a class at one of our local colleges or trying a new puzzle?

Again, congratulations on making it to your mid-70's with so few problems. However, this is the time to fearlessly look at your lifestyle to see if you've picked up any bad habits that you need to eliminate. You've done a great job so far, but don't be afraid to take your health to the next level.

Chapter 18

COLON CANCER SCREENING

Dr. Anne, I had an FOBT that was positive one year and negative the next. My doctors keep leaving town, but some doctors say I am fine while others say I need a colonoscopy. I am not fond of the idea of a mechanical object maneuvering through my innards. You should probably also know that my father had colon cancer. D from Independence

Dear D, Thank you for this excellent question, but the answer is going to require some background information first. FOBT is shorthand for Fecal Occult Blood Test. The fecal occult blood test determines "Is there hidden (or occult) blood in the feces (stool)?"

For those who don't know, a colonoscopy is the procedure during which the patient is mildly sedated and then a flexible scope is inserted into the rectum. On the front end of the scope there is a light and a video camera, a small pair of pincers that can be used to take a tiny biopsy, as well as a cautery loop for removal of polyps.

Colon cancer starts with a benign (meaning non-cancerous) polyp. If that polyp is left in place, over time it can transform on a cellular level and can eventually become a cancer. If we take the polyp out while it is benign, there is no opportunity for cancer. For this reason, the surgeon removes any polyps that are found during a colonoscopy. Even if the doctor finds polyps every time you have a colonoscopy, as long as the polyps are taken out, you should be fine.

Obviously, the colon must be completely cleared of any fecal material so that the doctor can see the walls of the colon. So, the night before the procedure, the doctor will prescribe a series of laxatives to clear the colon. This is called the "bowel prep." Many people feel that the bowel prep is the worst part of the whole procedure, and I agree that it's pretty miserable. But, what is actually worse is if you go through the bowel prep, but didn't do it thoroughly enough. In this case, the doctor either has to have you repeat the bowel prep and then re-scope, or he just says "incomplete prep," leaving you wondering if there was a problem that could not be seen. So, when it is time for a colonoscopy, don't skimp on the bowel prep!

We used to say that everyone over 50 should have a colonoscopy once every 10 years, or they could have a FOBT yearly and a sigmoidoscopy every 5 years. The sigmoidoscopy is just like a colonoscopy, but it only looks at the last 1/3 of the colon. This second option never made good sense to me. First you have to mess with your poop every year to get the FOBT and then you have to do a bowel prep every 5 years instead of every 10. In addition, the majority of colon cancers are in the ascending colon, which is not seen in the sigmoidoscopy. How is that better? Now the recommendation is that everyone start having colonoscopies every 10 years starting at age 45, or you can still do the yearly fobt plus the sigmoidoscopy.

Then, in about 2012, some brilliant person developed a more sensitive FOBT test called an "**immunochemical** fecal occult blood test," which can detect much more minute quantities of blood in the stool. The reason this is important is because polyps rarely bleed, they just "shed" a few red blood cells onto the stool.

Let me explain. The polyp cells are not normal colon cells. One of the abnormalities is in the basement membrane, which means that the cells don't hold together very well. Think of it like the mortar between bricks not working well. In addition, cancerous polyps actually secrete a hormone that stimulates the body to grow more blood vessels to the polyp so that it can get more than the normal share of nutrients through the blood. So you have an area with extra blood supply, and cells that don't hold together as tightly as they should. Then, as the stool moves through the colon, the polyp gets "rubbed" and it tends to shed fragments of red blood cells into the feces. The old FOBT test could not detect these tiny amounts of blood, but the immunochemical FOBT can.

So, we have changed our recommendation on cancer screening. Option 1 is still a colonoscopy every 10 years. Option 2 is to have the new immunochemical FOBT every year. If you have a negative immunochemical FOBT every year, we can be reasonably certain that you are colon cancer free. If you have a positive immunochemical FOBT, then you need to have a colonoscopy to go check things out. Of course, there are things that will cause the immunochemical FOBT to be positive that are not a cancer (we call this a false positive). Examples would be a bleeding ulcer, a bleeding hemorrhoid, etc. Obviously, if polyps are found, you will need a follow up colonoscopy sooner than 10 years.

Now, you asked, what if you have an immunochemical FOBT positive one year and you choose to ignore it. Then the next year you repeat it and it is negative. Well, then you are gambling that the positive test was a false positive. Hopefully, you had a bleeding hemorrhoid when you took the test. If you had an upper GI bleed at the time, things would have gone downhill fast so those can probably be eliminated as a possibility. But, in essence you are risking that you have a polyp that is intermittently shedding blood.

The fact that you have a first degree relative (that means mother, father, or siblings – not aunts, uncles, or grandparents) that had colon cancer makes me much more nervous. Many doctors feel that the immunochemical FOBT yearly should ONLY be an option for patients without significant risk factors. Having a first degree relative with a colon cancer history could be considered a significant risk factor. So, I have to ask, "What is your goal here?"

I have a friend who has this thing about the seat belts on airplanes. Every time she flies she leaves her seat belt unbuckled and covers it with her purse so the flight attendant can't see it. She says that she feels like she is somehow winning. I have another friend who refuses to disinfect his contact lenses, despite the strong recommendations of every eye doctor on earth. These are crazy behaviors! It is like playing Russian Roulette!

The doctor who says you need a colonoscopy is just trying to keep you healthy. Here is something else you should consider. Studies show that even the specialists who do colonoscopies every day, miss 15% of polyps. Holy smokes, if I had a parent who had colon cancer, I would be getting that scope as often as anyone recommended, so that I would increase my chances that they would find anything abnormal, and find it early. Colon cancer is nothing to mess around with. Colorectal cancer is the second leading cause of cancer death in the U.S. and of course the death rate increases with age.

Get the scope NOW and be assured that you are cancer free!

Chapter 19

WHAT ABOUT MY HIATAL HERNIA?

Dear Dr. Anne, I have been told that I have a hiatal hernia. Some doctors tell me that it is no big deal and I don't need to worry about it. Other doctors say that I will need surgery someday. I am confused and a little concerned and I was hoping to get more information. Can you help? Signed J, from Coffeyville.

Dear J, I hope that I can help. Let's start with some background. A hiatal hernia occurs when a part of the stomach has herniated (poked through) the diaphragm into the thorax (the chest cavity). About 10% of adults have hiatal hernias and the risk increases with age, obesity, being male, and if others in your family have had them. Having a hiatal hernia can increase your chances of having gastro-esophageal reflux disease, commonly abbreviated as GERD, and also known as heartburn (although it has nothing to do with your heart). From everything that I have learned in studying medicine, surgical repair is not usually required, but then again, I would not say that it is rarely done – more about the necessity of surgery below.

There are four types of hiatal hernias. I have provided a drawing of the stomach below that I hope helps as we talk about hiatal hernias. It also includes the names for the different parts of the stomach.

Hiatal Hernia

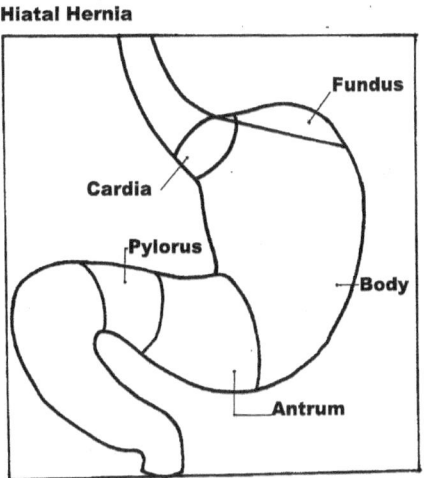

A Type I hiatal hernia is also called a sliding hernia and that is where the cardia (the very first part of the stomach) slips up above the diaphragm into the thorax – see images below. Ninety percent of all hiatal hernias are this type.

A Type II hiatal hernia is sometimes called a true or paraesophageal hernia. In this type the fundus (the top "humped" portion of the stomach) herniates through the diaphragm. These make up only 3% of hiatal hernias.

Type III hiatal hernias are sort of a combination of Type I and Type II. You can see below that both the cardia and the fundus have slipped up into the thorax.

And finally, Type IV hiatal hernias are the same as a Type III plus something else is also protruding into the chest cavity. In the picture below, the entire stomach is shown above the diaphragm, but it could be a section of small bowel, large bowel, or pancreas, etc.

Hiatal Hernia 2

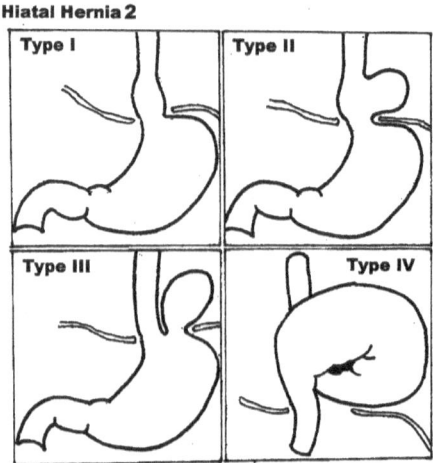

Any of these hernias can worsen with time. In other words, as you age, more tissue can migrate up into the thorax. Why? Well, darn it, just like our skin losing elasticity as we age, the same thing happens to pretty much all our tissues, including those tissues in our gut and our diaphragm. The older we get, the more our bellies grow, the more we cough or vomit (all of which increase the pressure under the diaphragm), the more likely it is for the "stuff" that should be below the diaphragm to get pushed up above the diaphragm.

So, when should we worry about our hiatal hernias? First, if you have a hiatal hernia and you have GERD, make sure that you are treating the GERD appropriately. The vast majority of GERD can be successfully treated with medication and lifestyle modifications. Talk to your doctor about the different medications for GERD, but lifestyle changes that can help with GERD are as follows:

(1) If you are overweight you need to lose some. Being in the obese category will make the GERD worse; even a 10% drop in weight will help dramatically.

(2) Always eat ONLY very small meals. It is fine to eat more frequently, even every 2 hours, but the amount must be small so that there is less food in the stomach (which will translate to less acid) pushing up into the esophagus.

(3) Never lie down on a full stomach. It is best to wait 3 hours after eating before you lie down so that the food has moved down past the stomach and cannot back up into the esophagus when you lie down.

(4) Try sleeping at an angle, to get a little help from gravity. For many people never lying flat helps control their GERD. So, use pillows or elevate the head of your bed on bricks.

(5) Stop smoking. Smoking is not directly associated with hiatal hernia formation, but smoking is associated with GERD and with loss of elasticity of all tissues. If you happen to have a hiatal hernia, and are a smoker, stopping smoking would greatly improve your life span as well as your daily health.

When is surgical repair of a hiatal hernia necessary? If you have a hiatal hernia and GERD, and have tried all of the other more conservative treatments for GERD (medical and lifestyle) and you are still having symptoms, then you should consider surgery.

The more obvious justification for surgery, is when whatever tissue has pushed up into the thorax is now causing other problems, like an obstruction; whether it is an obstruction of the stomach or of the small or large intestine, it doesn't matter. If you have a bowel obstruction, you have to have surgery, period, but this is not common. Rarer still, some hiatal hernias seem to be associated with other adverse events in the bowel like a volvulus. This is where a section of the large bowel flips over and causes a great deal of pain.

In general, let abdominal pain be your guide. If you have a hiatal hernia, but you are not in pain, then there is absolutely nothing to worry about. If you have a hiatal hernia and GERD, then you need to treat the GERD. If you have a hiatal hernia and GERD and you cannot get the GERD under control even after trying all the lifestyle modifications and multiple meds, then it is time to see a surgeon for a consultation.

I am glad you asked about this. There is absolutely no reason to worry and wonder about a health problem. Worrying adds to your underlying stress level and that is definitely NOT healthy. Knowledge is empowering. Acting on that knowledge relieves stress and adds confidence, peace of mind and hope. A life filled with peace and hope is a life with joyous possibilities.

Chapter 20

ARE THE FREE CANCER SCREENINGS WORTH IT?

Dear Dr. Anne, I have heard that there is going to be some free cancer screening in Indy on October 1st. Is this really worthwhile or just a way to get you hooked in to a new doctor? Signed L, from Independence.

Dear L, Thanks for writing. You heard correctly, free cancer screening is being offered by staff from KU Med Center, and sponsored by the Independence Masonic Lodge. It will be held at the Masonic Lodge, located at 2000 West Laurel, from 9:00 a.m. to noon.

Unfortunately, to answer your question, I have to start by asking one of you. Do you get regular, yearly checkups and cancer screening somewhere else, perhaps from your primary care provider (PCP)? If your PCP is very thorough, then you may not need to take advantage of this free screening. If, however, you either do not have a PCP or your PCP is constantly rushed like I was when I had a clinic, then this cancer screening is a great idea. After all, how often does your PCP have time to have you get totally naked and check your entire body for signs of skin cancer?

The screening that is being offered on October 1st, for both men and women, will include screening for skin cancer, oral cancer, prostate cancer, and osteoporosis. If you have ever been screened for skin cancer by a dermatologist, then you know that it is uncomfortably thorough. I had assumed that during this event, they would just be checking sun exposed areas like your face, neck, hands and arms. But, I have been told that there are going to be curtained exam areas and I am assuming you will disrobe.

If you are a smoker, or have a significant smoking history, or chew tobacco, then you definitely need to have someone checking your mouth yearly. If your PCP or your dentist are not getting that done, then you REALLY need to show up. Don't even think about missing this opportunity.

Medicare recommends that all men over 50 years old have screening for prostate cancer. You may recall that I addressed prostate screening in an earlier column. To reiterate, you don't have to have prostate cancer screening yearly, but you do need to have it. Although prostate cancer is much more prevalent in the 50's and 60's, it is by no means unheard of in the 40's, but as I said, Medicare won't cover it until you are over 50 years old. So while it is free, if I were male and over 40, I would show up! It is my understanding that they will have a private room where they will be screening with digital rectal exams. I know you guys are thrilled.

Although osteoporosis is not a cancer, it is a serious disease in the elderly and this screening will also be offered. All post-menopausal women (including those who have gone through surgical menopause) need to be checked for osteoporosis. Medicare will only pay for osteoporosis screening starting at age 65 so this is a great opportunity to get checked when you really need it and without cost. In addition, elderly men, and especially those who have low testosterone levels, should also be checked for osteoporosis.

It is important to note that you don't have to live in Indy to participate. I believe that screening is offered to anyone in the area. I also want to mention that every April, CRMC offers free screening for cervical cancer, skin cancer, and prostate cancer, both in Indy and in Coffeyville. It is highly likely that Labette Health and Wilson County Hospital, who also have offices in Indy, will also be offering cancer screening.

Don't overthink this; it is a great opportunity. So, just do it.

Chapter 21

THE NEW YORK TIMES ARTICLE ON THE SUGAR SCAM

Dear Dr. Anne, What do you make of the recent article in the New York Times about the sugar industry paying off Harvard researchers in the 60's? Signed, W from Independence.

Dear W, thank you, thank you, for writing in about this! I have been dying to talk about it.

For any readers who missed the article, you can Google it, but on September 12th, the New York Times published a surprising article. They had found irrefutable evidence that, in the 1960's, the sugar industry paid Harvard researchers to cover up the link that they had found between sugar and heart disease AND to shift the blame onto saturated fats instead. The article stated that most of the researchers have since passed away, but they were able to interview one man who was involved. Reading his response took my breath away. In response to the accusations, he said, "By today's standards, we behaved very badly." In my opinion, the truth should not change according to the social standards of the day and does not change whether the year is 1966 or 2016.

However, moving on to something more positive about this new information…this is great news, because it confirms what many doctors have been trying to do over the last 10-15 years. That is letting people know that a reasonable amount of fat in your diet will not kill you, but sugar will!

Please don't stop reading just because you have heard me run on about sugar in the past. In previous columns I was only addressing the connection between sugar and obesity and diabetes. But now, I can say with even more assurance that cutting out, or at least cutting down, on your sugar intake will reduce your risk of heart disease. That is HUGE! I am not saying it will be easy; it won't be. Remember sugar is addictive. It hits the same receptors in the brain that opium does. That is why you feel euphoric, at least for a couple of minutes, after eating candy. Did you know, that when a male infant is going to be circumcised, he is given a tiny vial of sugar water and most of the time, he won't even cry during the procedure?!

But there are so many really great sugar alternatives available today. Do you guys remember TAB? Now that stuff was vile. Today there are great alternatives and many of them are available at our local stores. Here's an example: Quest Protein Powder

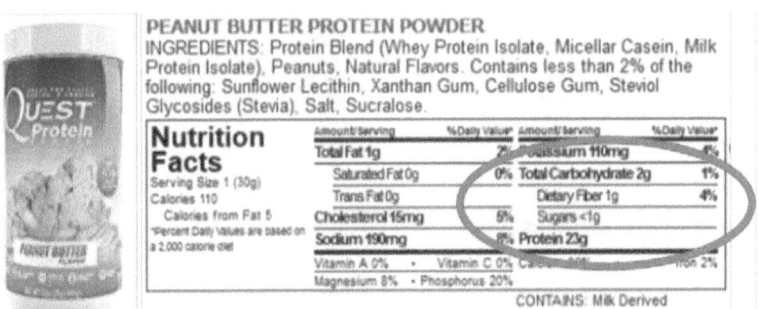

Now, let me explain why it is a great, healthier alternative to ice cream. First, it tastes great. Second, nutritionally it is also great. Let me show you how you can tell if it is nutritionally good for you. I circled the most important part of the nutritional label. Do you see

how "Dietary Fiber" and "Sugar" are indented underneath "Total Carbohydrate?" Dietary fiber is really about cleaning your colon. So any time you see "Dietary Fiber" you get to subtract that from the "Total Carbohydrate" number to get your "Net Carbohydrates" or your "Impact Carbohydrates." For maximizing your health and minimizing the negative impact of your sweet treat, you want as little sugar as possible, as few "Net Carbohydrates" as possible, and ideally a lot of protein, because it will help offset the flood of sugar into the blood stream, level your blood sugar and keep your energy level up. In the example above, there are two grams of total carbohydrates and we get to subtract one gram of dietary fiber. That means there is only one Net Carb or Impact Carb. And, to make things even better, there are 23 grams of protein! This is what you want; very little sugar, lowest possible number of "Net Carbs," and highest possible protein. This is a great option.

Here is another delicious example:

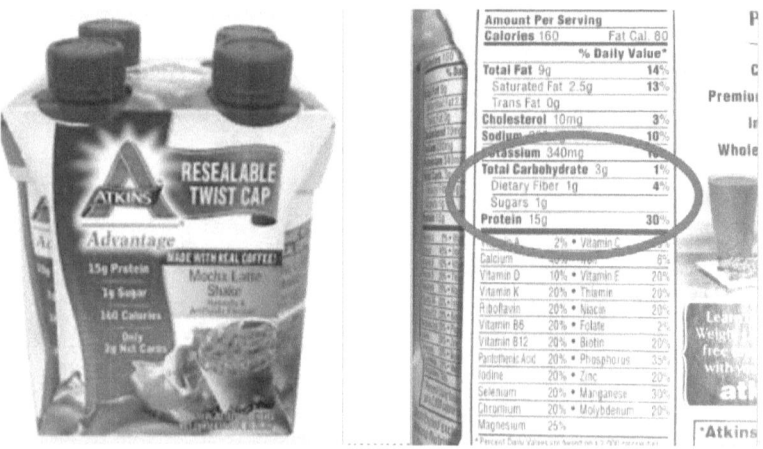

These shakes come in lots of yummy flavors, and they have very little sugar. But, let's review how many "Net Carbs" they have. The flavor in the picture of the nutritional info photo is "Mocha Latte" and the label shows three grams of total carbs and we get to subtract one gram of fiber, leaving a total of 2 grams of "Net Carbs" AND there are 15 grams of protein. Again, LOTS more protein than carbs, so it will not spike your blood sugar and there is only 1 gram of sugar, which is not enough to have a negative impact on your heart; at least as far as we know now.

If you forget how to calculate your net carbs, many healthy packages with show you.

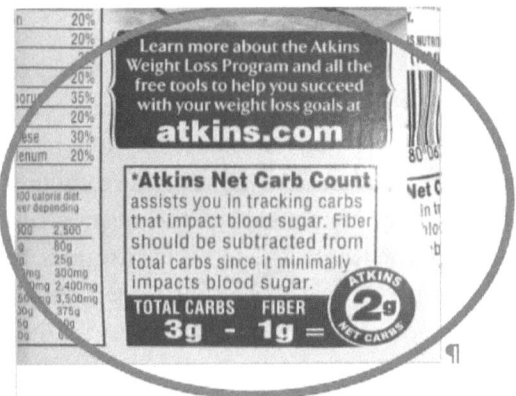

Now, there are many other brands, some are even better with more protein and are available at our local stores. But I am just trying to give you a couple of examples. At the same time, please don't get suckered in by products that say on the front that they are high protein or low sugar, but on the back, the nutritional information tells a very different story. For example, the Atkins Endulge Peanut Butter Cups:

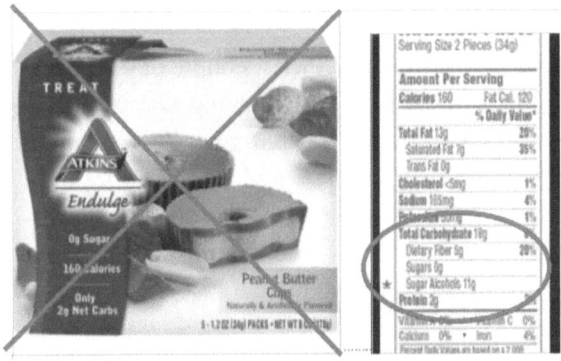

Now, here you can see that there are 18 grams of total carbohydrates and we subtract 5 grams of dietary fiber for a "Net Carbohydrate" count of 13 grams. Unfortunately, there are only 2 grams of protein. So, I would NOT eat these. But, looking closely you point out that there are ZERO grams of sugar, so why can't you eat this one as a healthy sweet treat? Well, you would be right that there is no sugar, but there are 11 grams of sugar alcohol.

We haven't had a chance to talk about sugar alcohols much, and there really isn't time here today, but there are many different sugar alcohols. Some have little or no impact on your blood sugar and others have a huge impact. We can talk more about that another time, but I stay away from most of the sugar alcohols. First, I haven't memorized the whole list, and I don't want to take the time to look up the impact of each one, but more importantly several of them are very strong laxatives. I promise, it is NOT, a pretty picture.

In summary, we now have new compelling information to encourage us to continue to minimize or even eliminate sugar from our daily intake. Recent polls showed that Kansas is the 7th most obese state in the union. But, we can change that! When you need a sweet treat there are some great alternatives out there that are readily available. But, as always, you must read the back of the package and NOT trust what is on the front of the package. Now you know how to do it.

The holidays are coming up. Pick a couple of days and let yourself splurge on those days, like Thanksgiving Day and Christmas day. But, please do NOT start your splurge at Neewollah and continue through the New Year! Come on Montgomery County, let's show the other counties of Kansas how this is done!

Chapter 22

RECOGNIZING MELANOMA

Dear Dr. Anne, I have a spot on my neck that my wife is saying I should mention to my doctor. How important is the whole skin cancer thing? I don't remember all the worry about skin cancer when I was a kid. Signed, B from Cherryvale.

Dear B., I am so glad that you asked that question; it is a big concern. So, let's go over the basics.

First and foremost, ABSOLUTELY YES, have your doctor look at ANY spots that you have that are **new**, or **growing**, or **changing**. Do not wait, do not pass Go, do not collect $200, just go to the doctor and have them check you out. It is true that most of the changes that we see on our skin as we age are just freckles, and moles, and warts, and age spots, and sun spots, and other completely benign (non-cancerous) "stuff" that just happens to us as we get older. But, again, spots that are **new**, or **growing**, or **changing** should be checked.

There are three major types of skin cancer: squamous cell, basal cell, and melanoma. Squamous cell and basal cell do not metastasize, that is the cancer cells won't migrate to another area of the body and start growing there. So, in general, they are not nearly as deadly. Melanoma is the most serious concern skin cancer, because it can be very aggressive and it can metastasize. However, there are cases where someone has let a squamous cell or a basal cell go crazy and grow and grow, until it eventually is a life threatening problem. So please do NOT put this off. It is so much easier to remove something when it is small instead of waiting until it is large, and you end up being disfigured. Please don't do that.

Here are the basics that everyone should know:
1) Fair haired, fair skinned, and red haired people are more at risk that darker skinned people.
2) However, just because your skin is dark, does NOT mean that you are immune. Anyone can get skin cancer regardless of your skin color.
3) Sunscreen and hats really do help. Enjoy the sun, but cover up and don't forget to put sunscreen on the top of your ears if you are only wearing a cap or a visor.
4) Skin that is constantly exposed to the sun, such as the face, neck, ears, hands and arms are where most skin cancers happen.
5) The argument that the benefits of spending a lot of time in the sun, which makes more vitamin D, outweigh the risk of skin cancer, does not hold water.
6) The logic that "one good sunburn early in the season will really jumpstart your tan" is crazy! Sunburns really are burns. If you want to tan, take it slowly.
7) Here are the basics of what you should be concerned about. ALL of us need to keep in mind the **"ABCDE"** of skin cancer screening.
8) **A stands for Asymmetry** – if one side of the spot looks different than the other side, then you need to have that spot checked out.
9) **B stands for Borders** – is the border smooth or irregular. A smooth border is more likely to be benign, but if the border is not smooth, then you need to have that spot checked out.

10) **C stands for Colors** – if there are multiple colors in the mole, then you need to have that spot checked.

11) **D stands for diameter** – If the diameter of the spot is greater than 6 mm, which is about the size of a pencil eraser, then you need to have that spot checked.

12) **E stands for Evolving** – Again, if you have a spot that is changing, then you need to have it checked out.

There are lots of examples of the ABC's of melanomas on the internet, so just google it for photos. Also, please notice that if any ONE of the ABCDE's are present, then you need to have it checked out. In addition, many doctors feel that there should be a "**T**" added to the ABCDEs and that the "**T**" would stand for **texture**. Benign lesions can be raised and look like they are "stuck on," but a flat, rough spot can be a concern.

The ABCDEs are taught in med schools, this is how new doctors are trained to recognize skin cancer. Past this basic knowledge, the only thing that helps the doctor is experience; looking at lots and lots of skin lesions.

If you have a spot and the doctor is not absolutely confident that it is benign, then ask for a biopsy. Yes, the numbing medicine hurts for a few moments, but a biopsy will tell you if there is a problem. But, again, please don't wait. If you have a new, or changing spot, or a spot that fits any of the ABCDEs then go in NOW and have it checked.

Chapter 23

KNOW A STROKE WHEN YOU SEE IT

Dear Dr. Anne, I've heard that if someone is having a stroke, they need to be rushed to the ER. So, I have two questions. First, what's the hurry? And second, if I really do need to hurry so much, how do I know when someone is having a stroke? Signed L, from Cherryvale.

Dear L, these are great questions and I am so glad that you asked me to address them. As usual, let's start with some basics.

A stroke occurs when blood supply to the brain is inappropriately altered. There are basically two types of strokes; *Ischemic*, where there is not enough blood supply to a particular part of the brain, and *Hemorrhagic*, where there is a bleed in a particular part of the brain. Ischemic strokes are much more common than hemorrhagic strokes; most studies show that about 85% of strokes are ischemic and only 15% are from a hemorrhage. However, it is also important to know that ischemic strokes can spontaneously convert to hemorrhagic strokes, especially in the first 24 hours.

If someone comes to the ER and has signs of a stroke, two things need to happen very quickly; first the blood sugar needs to be checked. Although most of the time having a very low blood sugar makes you to feel sweaty and shaky, it can also cause symptoms that completely mimic those of a stroke. The second thing that needs to happen is a CT scan of the head to see if there is a bleed in the brain. Please notice that the CT will ONLY tell us if there is a hemorrhagic stroke. It cannot tell us if there is a new ischemic stroke.

So, you might ask, "Why get a CT scan if it will only diagnose 15% of strokes?" And, I say, "Excellent question!" A stroke is actually diagnosed based on symptoms, not on what is seen on a scan. An MRI can usually, but not always, show an ischemic stroke. But, there are two drawbacks to an MRI. The first is that they take a long time and the second problem is that you won't always see the stroke with an MRI either in the very early stages or if it is very small.

On the other hand, CT's are fast, which leads us to the "What's the hurry?" part of your question. If the stroke is ischemic AND if the patient meets certain criterion AND if we are within **4.5 hours of the onset of the symptoms**, then we can give a drug that helps break-up the clot that is blocking the blood flow to the brain. If the blood supply can be restored quickly, then the stroke will resolve. And, in many cases, the symptoms simply melt away! It is pretty darn miraculous. But, if it takes 4 hours to get the MRI then we have usually wasted too much time and can no longer give the clot busting drug. There are also new procedures to remove the clots, but again, we have to hurry, because any cells that aren't getting appropriate blood supply are dying. Currently, we cannot do the retrieval of clots here in Montgomery County, but we can get that done in Bartlesville.

Now, that phrase about "if the patients meets certain criterion" is important and rather extensive. Think about this. If you are the doctor, and you are considering giving this patient a drug that will break up any blood clot no matter how tiny and no matter where it is in the body, you could be putting them at great risk of bleeding inappropriately. So the patient can't have had a recent surgery, can't have a genetic clotting problem, can't be on blood thinners, and the list goes on. For a long time we could not give the clot busting drug to anyone over 80 years old.

The clot busting drug is marvelous, but it also dramatically increases the chance that the ischemic stroke will spontaneously change to a hemorrhagic stroke. A small ischemic stroke can be survived and depending on where the stroke is in the brain, the patient may have minimal deficits afterward. But, if that small ischemic stroke converts to a hemorrhagic stroke because I gave a drug that breaks up any clots, the results could be devastating. Of course, we doctors take that very seriously. Hence, giving this drug is not always an easy decision, but the time window can be a deal breaker. If the patient comes in and has been having symptoms for 24 hours, we are outside the 4.5 hour window of opportunity.

Why is the time factor such a big deal? Again, if there is an area of the body that has not been getting blood for hours, then the tissue is essentially dead and flooding it with blood will not help. That is why we have a time window on this drug, which is why we need you to hurry and get to the ER as quickly as possible.

So, let's talk about recognizing stroke symptoms. Most of the time, stroke symptoms will be ONE SIDED. In general, the left side of the brain controls the right side of the body and the right side of the brain controls the left side of the body. So a clot on the right side of the brain will affect the left side of the body and vice versa. And, USUALLY, but not ALWAYS the symptoms come on SUDDENLY. There is a pneumonic that will help, it is F.A.S.T. If you notice sudden onset changes, then you should consider the possibility of a stroke and do the following:

F stands for Face. Ask them to smile. If one side of the **face** is drooping, go to the ER.

A stands for Arms. Ask them to hold both **arms** out straight in front of them. If one arm drifts down after a few seconds, go to the ER.

S stands for Speech. Ask them to repeat a phrase, like, "No if's and's or but's" or "Don't cry over spilled milk." If their **speech** is slurred or the words aren't right, go to the ER.

T stands for Time. This is just a reminder that time is important.

In addition, I would like to add **Balance**. If suddenly, they are falling and cannot walk, go to the ER. And, finally, if they have a sudden terrible **Headache**, unlike any headache that they have ever had before, please go to the ER.

There are a lot of things that can cause headaches, balance problems, falling, and confusion, so when you get to the ER, the doctor may be doing other work up besides the work up for stroke. The point is to get your loved one to the ER quickly when you notice a problem, so that the work up can begin and if the clot busting drug is called for, we can use this miraculous drug to restore function.

Chapter 24

URINARY RETENTION IN MEN

Dear Dr. Anne, I am a 59 year old man and I have noticed that when I urinate, it takes about twice as long as it did when I was 20. Do I need to be concerned? Signed G, from Independence.

Dear G., yours is an interesting question. There are several things that could be going on.

Scenario 1: The first thing that a doctor checks on when a man of your age reports changes in his urination is to ask what medications you are taking. Many meds can cause urinary retention; even over the counter meds like some antihistamines. So, first check any medication that you are taking to see whether urinary retention is a possible adverse side effect.

Scenario 2: As men age, their prostate gland will continue to grow as long as they have testosterone. I have included a graph showing the average testosterone level of men over a lifetime. You can see that although the level drops steadily through the years, you will still have significant testosterone between ages 80 and 100.

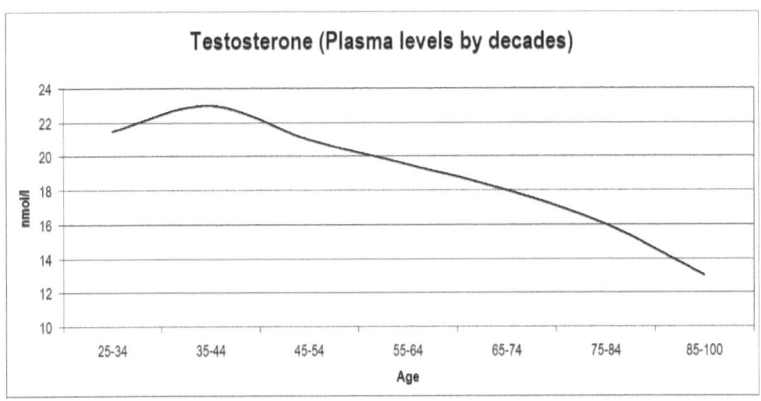

This means that your prostate will continue to grow essentially all your life. Unfortunately, your urethra, which is the tube that drains the urine from the bladder, is surrounded by the prostate. So, as the prostate grows it can crimp or compress the urethra. It is important to note that this is usually a non-cancerous increase in the size of the prostate.

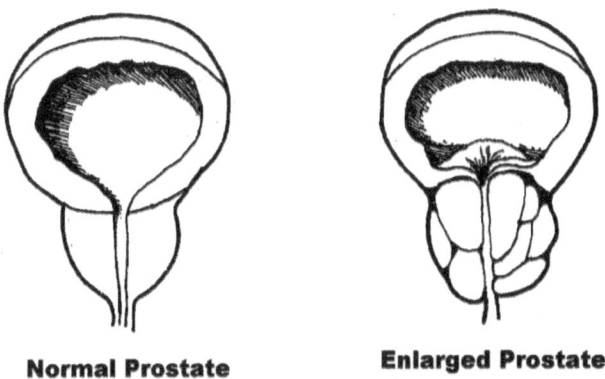

Normal Prostate   **Enlarged Prostate**

There are meds that can help with this problem. A very commonly prescribed med is finasteride, which blocks the production of testosterone. Another is tamsulosin, which relaxes the smooth muscles in the neck of the bladder and prostate. There are others, but most are related to one of these. If you have tried all the possible meds and nothing is working, there is a procedure called a

TURP, which stands for **T**rans **U**rethral **R**esection of the **P**rostate, where the urethra is basically reamed out.

Scenario 3: The third possibility is much less likely, but much more serious. This scenario is that there is a cancerous growth of the prostate that is blocking your urethra. Usually, prostate cancers are peripheral. In other words, they are most often on the outer portion of the prostate gland, but not always.

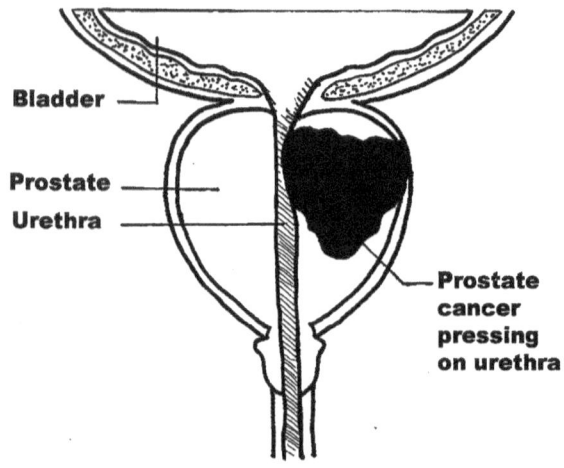

You may recall that we discussed prostate cancer screening in the past. However, if you are having symptoms, you need to have things checked. What symptoms am I talking about? Well, urinary retention, dribbling, frequent urination, or feeling that you are not able to fully empty your bladder. If these are present and you have not been checked in the last couple of years, then see your primary care provider or a urologist.

We have two urologists that serve Montgomery County. Dr. Howerter, in Coffeyville, is the only urologist that works in Montgomery County full time. I worked with him when I was with the Mercy Clinic and Hospital, but I work with him much more now that I am at the CRMC hospital, and I am confident in recommending him. Dr. Pai is a urologist in Parsons, but he drives to Independence twice a month to see patients. He used to see patients in the Mercy Clinic, but now has an office at the Labette Health Clinic in Independence. I can also recommend Dr. Pai.

Confounding Situation: It is not unusual for men to have a low serum (blood) testosterone level. What is confusing is that in spite of low testosterone, if they are getting hormone replacement, those men can still have an enlarged prostate, even if their testosterone level should remain on the low side. I don't have an answer to how this is possible, I just know that it is true.

So, the bottom line is that I would very much like for you to be seen by a urologist. As I mentioned above, we have two very good urologists that serve our county. I have worked with them both and have been impressed with their knowledge and their patient care. It is most likely a completely benign growth of your prostate, but it absolutely needs to be checked to make sure. At least have your PCP get a Prostate Specific Antigen blood test (PSA).

Chapter 25

WHAT ABOUT VITAMINS?

Dear Dr. Anne, My question is simple and straightforward and I am hoping that you can give me a simple and straightforward answer...Do I need to take vitamins or not? Signed, S from Coffeyville.

Dear S, We may actually be twin sisters separated at birth, because many times I have asked myself this very same question. And, I will try to make this very simple and straightforward. I grew up in a family where we took lots of vitamins, so as an adult, I have periodically wondered what is really necessary and what just makes me "feel" like I am taking care of my health.

The most simple and straightforward answer is that huge studies, with thousands of people in them, have shown that taking a multivitamin daily does NOT increase longevity. In other words, studies have shown that taking a daily multivitamin will not make you live any longer. However, that is only part of the story.

There are people who have difficulty absorbing the nutrients from the food they eat. Patients who have had any part of their small or large intestine removed or patients who have had bariatric surgery (for weight loss) are all at risk for malabsorption. These patients should really concentrate on eating as healthy a diet as possible, because their ability to absorb nutrients is reduced simply by the reduction of their gut length. Absorption of the nutrients in the food does not happen instantly. That is why our small intestine is 23 feet long. If you lose some of that, then the food may not stay in the intestine long enough to get all the nutrients out of it. In that case, supplements can increase the amount of those nutrients in your gut and increase the chance of you getting what you need.

Another group of patients that may need supplements are those with a very restricted diet. Whether the patient is just a picky eater, or their diet has been restricted for financial reasons, or their diet is restricted because many foods cause diarrhea, or gas, or heart burn, or whatever, these patients may also need supplements. Patients with Celiac, or Ulcerative Colitis, or Crohn's may also struggle to properly absorb nutrients.

Any menstruating female is at risk for iron deficiency anemia and should be taking iron supplements. It is true that iron supplements can cause constipation because it can bind with your food, so try taking it on an empty stomach and see if that helps. With rare exceptions, **all** post-menopausal women and men over 60 need to be taking calcium and vitamin D every day. Anyone who is a daily alcohol drinker needs to take thiamine, vitamin B12 and folate (which is the same as folic acid). And certainly, if your eye doctor says you need specific vitamins, absolutely take what he or she recommends.

In general, there are times when supplements may help with quality of life, even if quantity of life doesn't change. For example, if you have really weak fingernails and you start taking a supplement for "Hair, Skin and Nails" and your fingernails get stronger, then I think you should probably keep taking it. You might not live any longer, but if the supplement made a noticeable difference, then you were probably lacking in something that the supplement is now supplying.

I do need to mention a couple points of caution. Many supplements contain magnesium stearate. It is apparently one of the "inactive" ingredients that is put in a lot of supplements. If you are struggling with diarrhea, stop taking ANY supplement that has magnesium stearate in it. **Anything** with magnesium in it can cause diarrhea. Think of "Milk of Magnesia" or "Magnesium Citrate." These are strong laxatives so be aware and read the labels carefully. Secondly, please do not overdo on anything. Never take more than the recommended dose.

What I recommend is to review what you are taking about every 6 months or so. Discuss it with your primary care provider. If you are taking something that you are not confident is really helping you, then stop taking it. You can always add it back. And most importantly, always remember that what you eat is critical to your health, and taking supplements won't make up for eating garbage. Eating right is far more important than taking supplements.

Chapter 26

IS IT A GIFT?

Well, I didn't get a question this week, so I am going to talk about something that I believe is absolutely critical to our future as a county, as a state, and as a nation. As we head into our holiday season, I want to encourage each of us to take a hard look at what we feed ourselves and our children.

When our kids were young, I remember struggling with trying to impress on them that "you are what you eat," and that a small amount of splurging is not a big deal, but daily sugar intake is not a good life style choice. Like most women, I LOVE to bake, and it is hugely gratifying to see someone's eyes light up when I set a plate of fresh baked cookies in front of them or pull a perfectly baked pie out of the oven. But, as I have watched more and more people of all ages struggle with the consequences of eating too much sugar, I had to take a hard look at what my baking was doing and whether I was truly giving someone a gift, or whether I am just feeding something in myself. After a ton of reflection, I decided that my baking was actually not a gift at all. It made me feel good and it made those I baked for feel good for a few minutes, but ultimately I was hurting both them and myself.

Obesity in our country is reaching a critical level and the saddest part of that picture is that it is starting younger and younger. If you are in your 50's or 60's and you are tired and achy all the time because your weight is over burdening your heart and lungs and your joints, you know that is awful. But, now think what it must be like for a 14 year old child to be dealing with the same issues. Take a look at the chart below. Childhood obesity is not just a problem in our country, but ours is the worst.

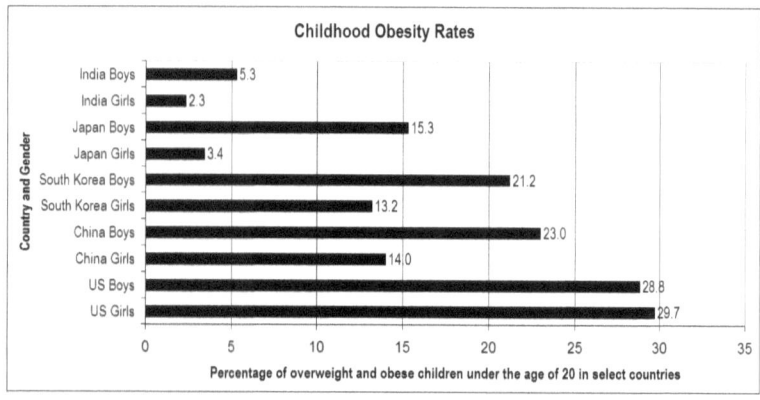

I know that if you have not seen the consequences of obesity you may not know why it is so very bad for you. But, let me try to explain what I see in the hospital every day. When someone is obese, they can function reasonably well for a while, but eventually the small muscles that move the rib cage can no longer lift the bulk of all of that weight that is acting like a heavy band around the chest cavity. When that happens, that person develops what is called obesity hypoventilation, where they just can't breathe, because they can't move their chest enough to take a deep breath. It is a form of restrictive lung disease. Look as the x-rays below. The first x-ray is a normal weight patient and the patient in the second x-ray is struggling with obesity. Try to imagine what it is going to feel like to try to lift all that weight to expand the lungs and take a deep breath.

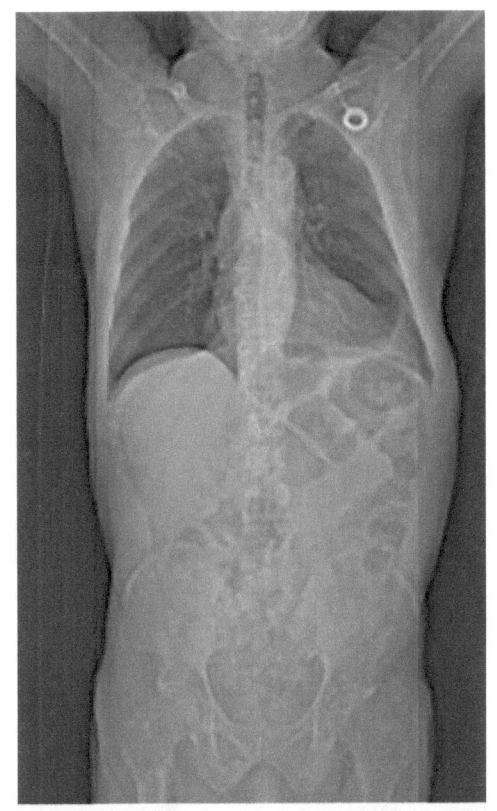

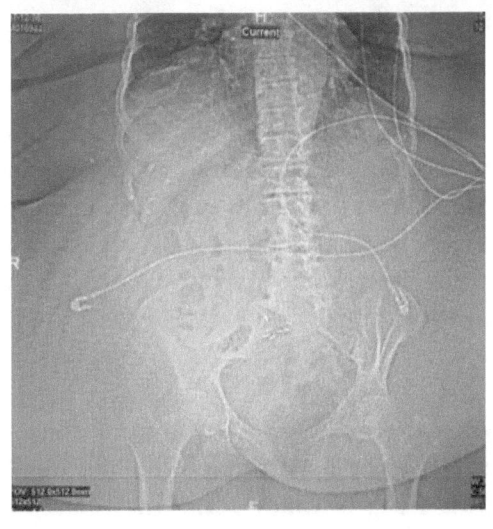

Another thing that happens is that the right side of the heart has to work really hard to push the blood into the lungs that can no longer expand because of the weight around them. Over time, this causes the right side of the heart to hypertrophy, which means it grows really thick. That might seem like a good thing at first, because we want our muscles to be big and strong, but it actually causes major problems. Just from looking at the picture below, you can see that the wall of right side of the heart has become big and the right ventricle (that is the lower chamber on the right) is dramatically reduced.

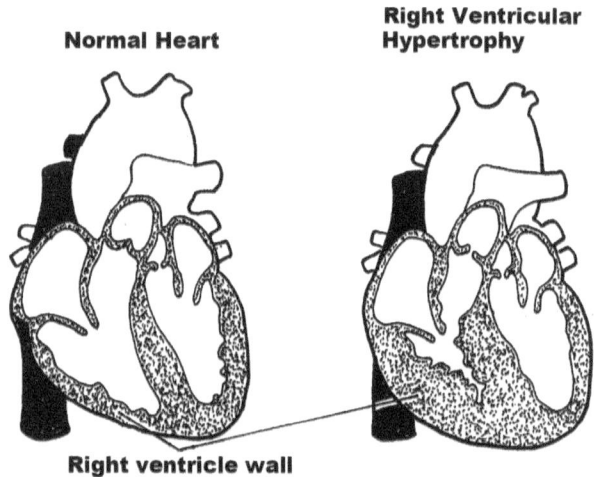

Normal Heart

Right Ventricular Hypertrophy

Right ventricle wall

Now, when the blood from the lower half of the body tries to get into the heart to be pumped into the lungs to get fresh oxygen, the right side of the heart is too stiff (it can't relax to accept the blood) and the chamber itself has gotten smaller. So, because the blood can't get into the heart, the fluid starts to back up into the legs. This is when we start to see the lower leg edema (swelling) that we see so often.

Please, as we head into the holiday season, don't give kids or yourself sweets at every opportunity. The kids don't need to be sent home with a bag of candy corn. They don't need a baggie with three iced Christmas cookies. A few years ago, one of my brothers and his family came to visit for Christmas. In preparation for their visit, I had bought chocolate kisses to put in bowls around the house to add what I thought was a festive touch. My brother and sister-in-law were very nice about it, but they said that they wouldn't come back with all the candy around. They didn't want to be tempted by it and they sure didn't want their kids tempted by it. It was an important lesson for me.

Last weekend was our Neewollah Grand Parade and I was thrilled to see that many of the floats had decided to give out beads instead of candy. And, as city crews and boy scouts cleaned up the trash, they told my husband that they picked up a ton of candy wrappers, but not a single string of beads.

When we were kids, one of my younger brothers was always asking for "a small cheap toy." Let's find other small gifts that we can give besides sugar. Southeast Kansas does NOT have to be the most obese part of Kansas. We can change this, but NOT if we keep feeding ourselves and those around us sugar.

Chapter 27

IS POSTURE MEDICALLY IMPORTANT?

Dear Dr. Anne, is posture important medically, or does it just make us look better? Signed L, from Independence.

I've got to tell you "L," my grandmother is tap dancing in heaven right now knowing that you asked that question. Lordy, she stayed on my case about standing up straight. There are several reasons why posture is important, but your spine's health is top on my list.

Maintaining a Healthy Spine: As a result of my grandmother's efforts, I did work at standing up straight, and always thought I had good posture. Then my neck "went out" one time in about 1994. I went to a chiropractor and he said something about my terrible posture. I was shocked and asked him to explain. He said that I was holding my head way too far forward. He went on to explain that the way to check your posture is to stand with your back to a wall. Your heels, your buttocks, your shoulders and your head should all touch the wall when you are standing up straight with good posture. See the illustration below.

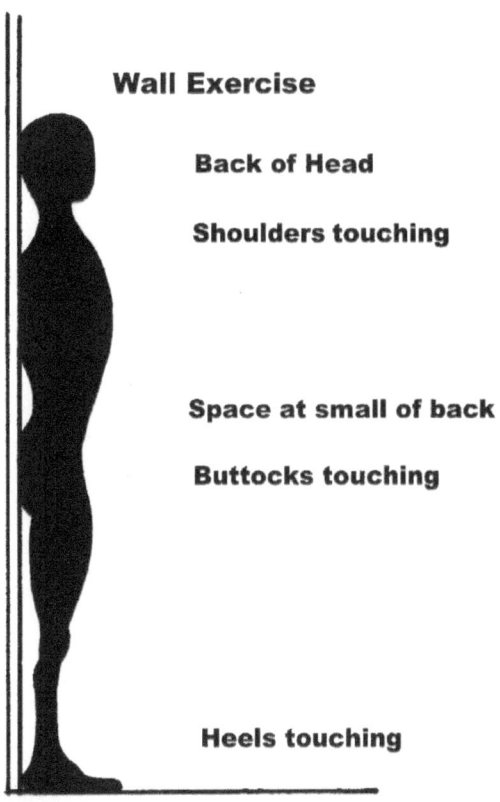

Wall Exercise

Back of Head

Shoulders touching

Space at small of back

Buttocks touching

Heels touching

I have to tell you that for the first year I tried the wall "exercise," the only way to make my head touch the wall was to look up at the ceiling!

My experience in adulthood has been that every few years I used to wake up with an extremely stiff and intensely painful neck or low back. That is what I meant in the previous paragraph when I said that my neck "went out." Sometimes I have been able to identify the event that caused the pain – like a strain from lifting something while twisting - but other times, I just seemed to have slept wrong. Either way, I usually got better with the help of a chiropractor and NSAIDs, within a couple of weeks with a neck problem, or within 4-6 weeks with a low back issue. While attending medical school, I learned a lot about preventing those episodes and why preventing them is more important than I realized. (I think the second question I ever addressed was on low back pain.)

When your spine is in pain like that, it is usually because a nerve is being pinched. The pinching of the nerve obviously causes pain, but also causes your body to send inflammatory chemicals to the area. Over time the body will actually lay down calcium, forming additional bone in that inflamed area. It's as if the body is trying to solidify that area so that it cannot be injured again. In the picture below, notice the bone that has formed connecting the vertebra. That "bone" formation will freeze the spine in that position.

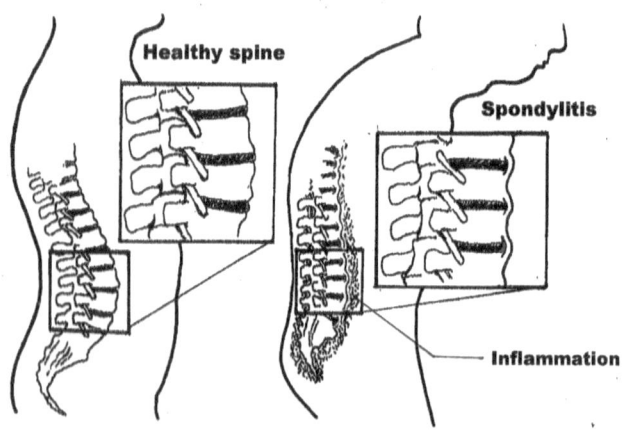

These "bone formation" changes can happen at any point along the spine and they obviously reduce your mobility and flexibility. They will also increase your chances of further injury because of the loss of flexibility. You can see that they will also cause continual strain on the ligaments, tendons, and muscles surrounding the spine. The **_only_** way to prevent these episodes is regular exercise and stretching, and chiropractic help when things are out of alignment.

Maintaining Healthy Joints: Much like the spine, any joint that is not aligned correctly will cause strain to the surrounding muscles, tendons and ligaments. Again, this causes inflammation and over time these joints will become painfully arthritic and eventually frozen. Equally important, many joints of the body have cartilage at the joint surface, which God designed to help cushion and lubricate the constant movement between the two bones. If the joint is not lined up correctly, then the cartilage can be worn away which causes much more wear and tear on the bones themselves.

Better Breathing: Try sitting in your chair right now with really bad posture – like you have been sitting at the computer for hours and your back is curved like a "C." Now, hold that position and without moving your spine, try to take the deepest breath that you can and notice how little air you are able to move through your lungs. Now, sit up very straight and take the deepest breath that you can. You can move about three times as much air when you are sitting up straight. So, imagine having your spine frozen in that very bent over position all the time, how are you ever going to take a deep breath? How will you have enough air to walk up a flight of stairs? This is one of the causes of Extra-thoracic Restrictive Lung Disease.

Improved Circulation and Digestion: Good posture allows the organs and the large blood vessels of the abdomen to be in the position that God intended for them. It opens the vessels and organs to allow the normal flow and functions of the entire digestive system. One problem that we have talked about in the past can be directly related to poor posture and that is GERD (Gastroesophageal Reflux Disease) – which is the same as heartburn.

Psychological Changes with Posture: There are other, less concrete reasons for good posture, but I believe that they are no less real. Good posture is thought to increase your confidence and your sense of wellbeing, possibly because you are getting better oxygen flow throughout the body and to the brain. Next time you are discouraged, force yourself to sit up very straight and take several deep breaths. Then reassess your situation. Just try it and see what you think. It costs you nothing and it may convince you that posture is every bit as important as my grandmother said that it was.

Chapter 28

FLU SHOTS, REALLY?

Dear Dr. Anne, are flu shots really important? Signed H, from Independence.

Dear H, what a great AND timely question. First let's talk a bit about the influenza virus. Influenza A and Influenza B viruses cause an acute respiratory illness that occurs every winter, in epidemic proportions, worldwide. Unfortunately, the influenza viruses can also cause pandemics. One of the worst pandemics in recorded history was the flu pandemic of 1918-1919 where an estimated 50-100 million people died of influenza. While that was 100 years ago, please don't think those days are completely in our past. The CDC estimates that between 36,000 and 41,000 Americans die every year as a result of the flu and its complications.

What is most remarkable about the influenza viruses is their ability to mutate very quickly. This makes it very difficult to vaccinate against. The US Center for Disease Control and Prevention (CDC) and the World Health Organization (WHO) track influenza virus isolates weekly and together form a database called FluNet. This database is an attempt to track the mutation of the influenza virus throughout the year, so that the CDC and the WHO can formulate a vaccine that they hope will cover the mutations that are going to take place for the coming season. Clearly, some years they do better than other years at predicting what the influenza viruses will do to try to get around your body's natural immune system. What a responsibility! I don't know about you, but that is a job that I would NOT like to have.

In addition to not contributing to a possible pandemic, another reason to get the flu shot is that there are very few antivirals against the influenza viruses. Oseltamivir and Zanamivir are active against both influenza A and B. Amantadine and Rimantadine are active only against influenza A and there has been a dramatic increase in resistance to these two drugs, so the CDC is recommending that these two not be given. None of these will treat any of the greater than 200 "common cold" producing viruses.

For Oseltamivir and Zanamivir, they must be given within 48 hours of onset of symptoms, which is difficult – once symptoms start it can be hard to get into the doctor and be tested for influenza within 48 hours of onset. Furthermore, they do not cure the flu, but can only shorten its duration by a few days. And, unfortunately, they are expensive, so between the 48 hour window, the expense, and the fact that they will only shorten and not cure the "flu," I actually rarely get to prescribe them. The exception to that is in hospitalized patients. Basically, if a patient is sick enough with the flu that they need to be hospitalized, then it is appropriate to give them Oseltamivir even if they are outside the 48 hour window.

Back to the whole vaccination question, there is a term that I need to introduce called "herd immunity." Basically, herd immunity means that if most of the population has been immunized, those that haven't are less likely to be exposed to the disease, because there is just not much of the disease around. The problem with relying on "herd immunity" is that more and more people are saying "no thank-you" to vaccinations, so those that are not vaccinated are going to be at greater risk. In fact, the increase in the number of people declining the flu vaccine, increases the risk of the yearly epidemic turning into another pandemic.

Let's be clear here. We doctors are very committed to "autonomy," which means that the patient gets to make their own health care decisions. So, if you don't want the flu shot, then I am going to say, "OK." There are people in my own family, whom I respect and love dearly, who have refused a flu shot for years. But, I get a flu shot every year, as do most all doctors and health care professionals. Doctors give their families a flu shot. Do I ever get sick? Of course, but I still recommend the flu vaccine to everyone over 6 months of age.

Chapter 29

YES, FLU SHOTS, REALLY!

Dear Dr. Anne, Last week you said that I DO need to get a flu shot, but every time I get a flu shot, I get the flu! Please address this! Signed P, from Independence.

Dear P, I don't blame you for being frustrated, but let me try to explain.

In general, there are two kinds of vaccines, (1) **inactivated vaccines,** and (2) **live-attenuated vaccines**. Inactivated vaccines are made from pieces of the pathogen (either a virus or bacteria). In the case of inactivated flu vaccines, there are trivalent and quadrivalent vaccines. That just means that there are pieces of either three influenza viruses or four influenza viruses added together to make the vaccine. When you are given the vaccine, your body recognizes the pieces of the viruses as foreign and develops antibodies to those shapes. In the months that follow, if your body's immune system encounters one of those shapes again (meaning you have been exposed to the flu virus), it will already have an antibody made to fit it. Once your immune system has attached an antibody to a foreign object, like a virus, then your body can destroy it.

The inactivated influenza vaccines are called Fluzone vaccines. As many of you know there is a standard dose and a high dose.

The standard dose Fluzone is recommended for EVERYONE between 6 months and 64 years of age. The high dose Fluzone is recommended for those individuals that are 65 and older.

Live-attenuated vaccines are made of weakened viruses (or bacteria). It is not just a piece of the pathogen, it is the whole virus or bacteria, but it has been modified so that you will be able to make antibodies without getting the illness. Theoretically, these vaccines will produce a stronger, more potent and protective immune response than the inactivated vaccines.

The big assumption is that you have a good immune system. And, most people do. However, as medical knowledge has expanded, so have the number of people with compromised immune systems. When we think of those with compromised immune systems, we always think of HIV patients first, but the number of cancer patients, transplant patients, and those on a whole host of new drugs used to treat rheumatologic and autoimmune disease has dramatically increased the number of patients with compromised immune systems.

The FluMist is given intra-nasally (a mist into the nose – not an injection). It is the live-attenuated influenza vaccine, and it is a quadrivalent vaccine. It is not available every year. But, clearly, its use is more limited, since you cannot have any immune issues and you cannot be over 50 years old.

So, can you get the "flu" from the flu vaccine? Well, it depends. First, if you have gotten an inactivated, intra-muscular injection, then the answer is actually "no." But, you can get sick! Just like an infant can have a fever after getting a vaccine. Your body is recognizing that vaccine as a foreign object. Your body does NOT like it. Foreign objects are NOT supposed to be inside us! Your body is supposed to react. You want it to react. It is more pleasant for us if there is no inflammatory response, but we really need the body to react and make antibodies, so that we can fight off the flu when we are exposed.

If you received the intranasal FluMist, that is a live-attenuated vaccine, AND if you have a compromised immune system, then yes, you could get the flu from the vaccine.

A question you might ask is, "How can I tell the flu, from the inflammatory response that you are talking about?" That is another great question and unfortunately, there is no definitive answer, but the inflammatory response is more like having a cold. So, below I have listed the signs and symptoms of the flu versus a cold. (Just because it is a fascinating tid-bit, over 200 different viruses have been identified that can cause "the common cold." Most of us can attest that some are common and some are fierce.)

Influenza Virus Symptoms	Cold Virus Symptoms
can have a sudden onset	rarely has a sudden onset
includes fever and chills	rarely includes fever and chills
fever will be 101 and over	if there is a fever, it will be lower
headache is common	can have headache
congestion will be severe	congestion is present
cough often produces severe chest pain	cough can produce chest pain
runny nose with thick phlegm	runny nose will start watery and then thicken
fatigue will be severe and can last 2-3 weeks	fatigue can be present and will last 3-7 days
illness lasts for 10-14 days	illness lasts 7-10 days
cough can linger for 6-8 weeks	cough can linger for 4-6 weeks

The only way to absolutely know that you have the flu is to be tested. That is usually done with a nose swab for the influenza antigen.

To wrap things up, the inactivated flu vaccines can cause an inflammatory response that feels like a cold, but they cannot cause the "flu." The live-attenuated flu vaccines can cause the "flu" **if** your immune system is compromised. However, these vaccines are much less common. Hope this helps.

Chapter 30

TREATING UPPER RESPIRATORY INFECTIONS

Dear Dr. Anne, when I go to see my doctor with a runny nose, sore throat, cough, and congestion, why won't my doctor give me an antibiotic? Signed A, from Independence.

Dear A, this is such a great question. When someone comes into a doctor's clinic with symptoms of cough, sore throat, congestion, etc. the doctor has to try to determine whether the symptoms are caused by allergies, a bacterial infection, or a viral infection - and if it is a viral infection, is it the "flu" or a "cold?" This has to happen, because the treatment for each of those is different. Unfortunately, it is not always clear what is causing the symptoms, because the symptoms overlap.

Allergies: Allergies will often cause watery or itchy eyes, runny nose, and usually have clear discharge either from the nose or the eyes, or both. Allergic reactions can make the nose feel like it is tight and swollen or bigger than usual. Sometimes patients say that it feels like their noses are blooming or about to explode. The roof of the mouth may itch. There is usually a lot of sneezing, but there can also be cough, because there is usually a lot of discharge running down the back of the throat, which triggers the cough. Allergies are treated with (1) avoidance of the allergen when possible, (2) antihistamines and leukotriene inhibitors, (3) decongestants, and sometimes (4) steroids.

But, medicine is complicated. You can also have an allergic reaction to a toxin produced by a cold virus. Or, you could be dealing with allergies and then get an infection from a virus or a bacteria on top of the allergy exacerbation.

Viral Infections: The vast majority (like over 90%) of upper respiratory infections are viral. Last week we talked about influenza and "colds" and how they present. You may also recall that we do have a couple of antivirals that can help shorten the duration of influenza (usually it will shorten the illness from 14 days to 10 days), but not cure it. Again, these drugs have to be given within the first 48 hours of onset, or they are not effective. And, unfortunately, these anti-viral drugs are quite expensive.

Again from last week, there are over 200 viruses that cause a "cold" and we have no cure for *any* of them. We can only treat the symptoms of a "cold" using – antihistamines, decongestants, acetaminophen, cough suppressants, additional fluids and above all, rest.

But, again, medicine is complicated and a viral infection can weaken your immune system and then a bacterial infection can settle in. The doctor may say, "This sounds viral to me. Let's give it a few days and see if you start to feel better with supportive care (like fluids, rest, antihistamines, decongestants, etc.). But, if you start to get worse, then come back in." The doctor is thinking that you have a "cold" and that an antibiotic won't treat a cold. A cold usually lasts about 7 to 10 days, but the worst of the illness will be days 2 through 6 and it should be tapering off after that. If day 6 or 7 are worse than day 4 and 5 then you may be getting a bacterial infection on top of the viral infection, and an antibiotic *will* help.

Bacterial Infections: Everyone is familiar with ear infections and "strep throat", which are both bacterial infections, but bronchitis, laryngitis, and pneumonia can all be either viral or bacterial. If the infection is bacterial, then antibiotics *MAY* help. I say the big "*MAY*" because there is a good deal of research that shows that in a majority of cases, ear infections get better on their own without antibiotics.

In general, if you present to your doctor with acute respiratory symptoms that have been present for less than a week and you are still able to be up and moving around and going to work, then you most likely have a viral infection and the doctor should *not* prescribe an antibiotic. If, on the other hand, you have had the symptoms for 7 days and in spite of staying in bed, you still have fever and feel terrible, then the doctor should prescribe an antibiotic, because if it was viral, you should be getting a bit better, unless it is the flu.

There is so much more I could say, but the bottom line is that antibiotics will ONLY help with a bacterial infection. And, again, the vast majority of upper respiratory infections are caused by viruses, which means that an antibiotic will NOT help.

Moreover, taking an antibiotic when you don't need it *can* cause a great deal of harm. How about I explain that next week?

Chapter 31

WHY SO STINGY WITH ANTIBIOTICS?

Last week we talked about all kinds of respiratory infections, both viral and bacterial, and when it is appropriate to take an antibiotic and when it is not. The question I'm typically asked next is, "Why not just give the antibiotic to cover all possibilities?" Today, I am going to try to answer that question.

I promise, doctors love to write prescriptions and we really love to make our patients happy. So, if I could just write a prescription for a course of antibiotics for anyone that it may help, I would. But, you have to remember that ALL medications have side effects. Heck, if you are taking a baby aspirin every day (81 mg) you have to stop taking it five days before having surgery because it "disables" your platelets, which means your blood won't clot well. So, the question really is, "What are the adverse side effects of antibiotic use, and in particular, the overuse of antibiotics?"

Yeast Infections: If you have never had a yeast infection, then count your blessings. Antibiotics are notorious for wiping out the normal "friendly flora" of the vaginal canal and opening up the opportunity for yeast to go crazy. This causes intense itching and burning in that area and sometimes a thick discharge as well. Overall, not a fun experience. If the antibiotic is treating a systemic illness, then it is worth the risk. But if the antibiotic is "just in case there is a bacterial component to this illness" then it is not.

Clostridium Difficile: A Clostridium Difficile infection, often called a "C-Diff Infection" or just "C-Diff," is a disruption of the "friendly flora" of the intestines. Many of us have some "C-Diff" bacteria hanging out in our intestines all the time. The amount of C-Diff is controlled by our "friendly flora." Unfortunately, antibiotics can wipe out the "friendly flora" and allow an overgrowth of the clostridium difficile bacteria, which causes a severe watery diarrhea. Usually, we can prescribe another antibiotic to clear it up; however, that is not always the case. C-Diff is occasionally known to cause a severe systemic illness with a very serious complication called Toxic Megacolon, where the large intestine can rupture. I don't think I need to explain why that's a bad thing.

Much more common are cases in which we just can't clear the C-Diff infection and the patient struggles for weeks or months with profuse watery diarrhea. In the worst cases, the only thing that has been shown to cure a recurrent C-Diff infection is a fecal transplant. Yes, you read that right; how horrifying is that? Someone else's fecal material is liquefied and run through a tube down the patient's nose and into the intestines to re-populate the friendly flora. And no, it is not sterilized, because that would kill the "friendly flora." Obviously, this is a situation that we doctors desperately try to avoid.

To make the situation even worse, not everyone has clostridium difficile in their gut. Those that don't are at great risk if they are exposed to even a little bit. C-Diff is extremely contagious and there is no hand sanitizer that will kill it. A good long scrub with soap and water is the only way to keep from passing it on. Again, **if** C-Diff infections were a rare complication of antibiotic use, then it would be different, but C-Diff is not rare. I see it often and so do most health professionals.

The Development of Resistant Bacteria: The problem with taking antibiotics when you don't need them is that, just like the influenza viruses we talked about two weeks ago, bacteria are constantly changing to try to protect themselves from antibiotics. Remember, bacteria are just like any other living creature. Some humans are stronger than others, some are more athletic, some are smarter, etc. When someone has a bacterial infection, that population of bacteria is similar in that individual "bugs" are stronger than others, and some can adapt to insult or injury better than others. When that person takes an antibiotic, the weak bacteria in their system will be killed, but those that are not as sensitive to the antibiotic, can continue to reproduce and develop resistance. So if we take antibiotics when we don't need them, we are predisposing ourselves to resistant bacteria.

This is what is causing the "super bugs" that you have heard about in the news. "Super Bugs" can cause untreatable infections that are becoming more and more prevalent. Everyone has heard of MRSA (which stands for methicillin resistant staphylococcus aureus), and pseudomonas (pseudomonas aeruginosa). But, there are actually many others that are even more difficult to treat.

Resistant bacteria, or "super bugs," are a huge concern among doctors. I know that when I had a clinic at Mercy, a couple of my patients were very angry with me, because they felt that I was being "stingy" with antibiotics. And I really do understand your frustration. As a doctor, when I have a bad cold, even knowing that it is viral, I am still tempted to take an antibiotic. The thing that stops me is the thought of resistant "super bugs," profuse watery diarrhea, an exploding colon, and an itchy, burning v-jj!

Chapter 32

HORMONE REPLACEMENT THERAPY FOR WOMEN

Dear Dr. Anne, Is it safe for women to take postmenopausal hormone replacement? Signed F from Independence.

Dear F., I like your question. It is clear and concise. Unfortunately the answer to whether or not Hormone Replacement Therapy (HRT) is safe is not quite as clear, and depends on the patient.

First, and most importantly, estrogen increases the risk of blood clots. So, if you have any other risk factors for blood clots, then hormone replacement therapy is NOT safe for you. Things that increase your risk of clotting are:
1) Daily Smoking – whether tobacco or marijuana
2) Obesity
3) A history of a previous stroke
4) A history of a previous blood clot
5) A current cancer of any kind
6) A genetic condition that increases the risk of clotting
7) Previous or current history of liver disease

A previous history of breast cancer does not necessarily increase your risk of clotting, but it does mean that HRT is not safe for you.

Secondly, it depends on how long ago you went through menopause. If you are somewhere between 47 and 52 years old and your periods are becoming infrequent, or if you are in your early to mid 50's and have recently stopped menstruating, then this is a good time to start HRT. However, if you stopped having periods 10 years ago, then it is too late to start HRT – studies have shown that reintroducing estrogen after you have been without it for several years definitely increases the risk of clotting – which can cause a stroke.

Next, we have to talk about **natural** menopause versus **surgical** menopause. If you have gone through surgical menopause (meaning you had a hysterectomy), then you have it easy and you can take estrogen without progesterone. You should start HRT soon after your surgery and stay on it until you feel like tapering off. That can be in your 50's or 60's, but you don't want to be pushing 80 and still be on HRT. Many of us who have had hysterectomies and are on HRT dread the thought of getting off, but we must do it at some point.

Unfortunately, if you still have your uterus you can ONLY use a combination of estrogen with progesterone. This is because estrogen stimulates uterine growth and unopposed uterine growth will cause uterine/endometrial cancer = "No Bueno."

The addition of progesterone causes two other problems. First, progesterone is the hormone that causes that awful premenstrual syndrome that we all struggle (or struggled) with for the few days just before our periods – the combination of extreme irritability and tearfulness. Lordy, sometimes I look back and I can't believe my husband stayed with me. Many times I just wasn't rational. Many post-menopausal women start on a combination of estrogen and progesterone and they just can't tolerate the progesterone.

More importantly, estrogen with progesterone has been shown to slightly increase the risk of breast cancer **IF** it is taken for **more than 5 years**. (If you are into statistics, it is an increase in the Relative Risk between 1.3 and 1.6 depending on which study you are reading – but remember, that an increase in Relative Risk is less than an increase in Absolute Risk – too much to explain here.) For most of us, even a small increase in cancer risk is not acceptable.

However, as I've said before, doctors in this country take patient autonomy very seriously. So, if you are a post-menopausal woman on combination HRT and you want to take that for more than 5 years, you can. The doctor will just document that he or she has warned you of the additional risks. But, if you end up getting breast cancer as a result continuing your HRT longer than 5 years, it would just be bad form to sue your doc.

If your symptoms are mostly vaginal, estrogen creams or the estrogen ring are effective, and in the short term (5 years of use), there have been no increases in the incidence of uterine cancer. But, we have no long term studies at this point.

For the loss of libido that comes with menopause, we used to add a very low dose of testosterone to the estrogen replacement. However, that is no longer recommended and there are no oral prescriptions that I can find to prescribe. There are still some bio-identical hormone replacement products available that include testosterone. Amazingly, we have one locally. That is Oswego Drug, in Oswego, Kansas. Your primary care provider can prescribe any combination of estrogen, progesterone, and testosterone that fits your needs best. Just be careful, a little testosterone can greatly improve your sex life, but even a little bit can cause acne and unwanted hair growth – and I don't mean on your head!

So, I am sorry to say, that the answer to your question is, "It depends." But, the good news is that even if HRT is not safe for you, we have other things that we can prescribe, which have been shown to help with those frustrating post-menopausal symptoms. How about we discuss those next week? And, by the way, these questions are great, keep them coming. Email me at IDRAskDrAnne@gmail.com.

Chapter 33

WHAT IF YOU CANNOT TAKE HORMONE REPLACEMENT THERAPY?

If you remember, last week we talked about post-menopause hormone replacement therapy (HRT) and whether or not it was safe. If you read through that column and found that, "No, it doesn't sound like I am a good candidate for post-menopausal HRT," then don't be discouraged. There are still alternatives that may help.

Just a quick review, HRT is too risky for those patients in the following situations:

1. Daily smoking
2. History of stroke
3. History of blood clots
4. History of breast cancer
5. Current cancer of any kind
6. A genetic condition that increases the risk of clotting
7. Previous or current history of liver disease
8. Obesity

If you have one of those, HRT is not a great option for you.

Someone who had read last week's column asked me, "Why is obesity included in your list of things that make HRT too risky?" So, just briefly, let me explain. Estrogen increases the likelihood of clotting. And, peripheral fat makes estrogen constantly – weird, I know, and not intuitive. So, if you are quite a bit over your ideal body weight, then your estrogen level is already higher than ideal. If we add more estrogen to that, you are much more likely to have a clot. That puts you at high risk for deep vein thrombosis, pulmonary emboli, myocardial infarcts and stroke.

But, again, we have other options. I have paraphrased the following chart from the American Family Physician Journal, December 1, 2016 issue. All of the following will help treat the hot flashes, the irritability, the loss of concentration and some of these drugs MAY also help with the forgetfulness, others will almost certainly make forgetfulness worse. You may recognize many of these drugs, and if you do, you may notice that the dosages are, in some cases, lower than when they are prescribed for other reasons. In all cases, we try to use the lowest dose possible to treat symptoms, so that adverse side effects are minimized.

Generic/Brand Name	Dose (mg/day)	$/mo – generic (brand name)
Citalopram/Celexa	10 to 20	$10 ($231)
Clonidine/Catapres	0.1	$9 ($79)
Desvenlafaxine/Khedezla	100 to 150	$257 ($384)
Escitalopram/Lexapro	10 to 20	$13 ($256)
Gabapentin/Neurontin	900 to 2,400	$14 ($340)
Paroxetine Salt/Brisdelle	7.5	NA ($190)
Paroxetine/Paxil	10 to 20	$10 ($178)
Pregabalin/Lyrica	150 to 300	NA ($185)
Venlafaxine/Effexor XR	37.5 to 100	$17 ($300)

Obviously some of these are expensive. Gabapentin is the only one that I know of that is known to cause confusion, and I personally don't like doses above 900 mg daily if at all possible. And, none of these will help with the vaginal dryness and atrophy. But, you can use estrogen cream, or just a nice lubricant for that.

So, I hope that was helpful. We really do have a lot of options to make the menopause transition easier. Unfortunately, menopause symptoms can last a long time. I had an 85 year old patient who swore she was still having hot flashes, bummer. I would love to say that was impossible, but I went through surgical menopause 10 years ago, and even on HRT, I still have hot flashes. Ah, well. I don't have them as often as I used to and since we are in the season of hope, I am ever hopeful!

Chapter 34

CARPAL TUNNEL SYNDROME

Dear Dr. Anne, I have started to have some numbness in my right hand. Is this Carpal Tunnel and if it is, what do I do about it? Signed T, from Cherryvale

Dear T, it's possible that you do have Carpal Tunnel, but the numbness may have any of several causes, so the first thing that you need to do is see your primary care provider (PCP). But, let me see if I can give you some foundational understanding about Carpal Tunnel and what can be done about it.

Carpal Tunnel Syndrome (CTS) is the most common "entrapment neuropathy" of the upper extremities. "Entrapment neuropathy" means that there is pathology involving a nerve that is caused by that nerve being trapped, compressed or restricted. On the inside of your hand/wrist there is an area called the "carpal tunnel" and the median nerve and nine flexor tendons pass through it.

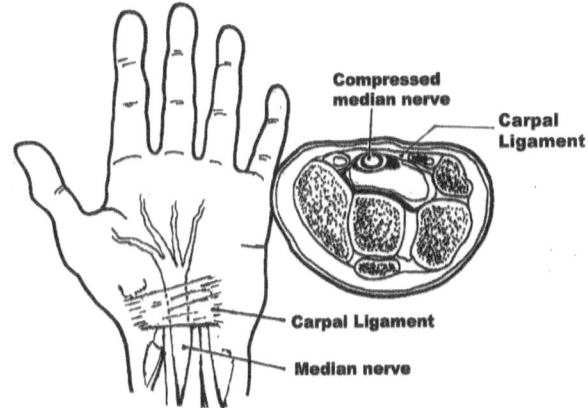

Anythng that causes chronic inflammation or swelling in that area can cause "Carpal Tunnel Syndrome" because it can cause the median nerve to be "compressed." Common risk factors are diabetes mellitus, obesity, hypothyroidism, pregnancy, and rheumatoid arthritis. Women are more likely to have CTS than men, and the prevalence increases with age. Forceful, repetitive hand exertions are also a risk factor.

The most common symptoms are pain or numbness in the distribution of the median nerve, which includes the palmar surface of the thumb, index and middle finger, and half of the ring finger. This palmar surface is shown as the dark area in the photo below.

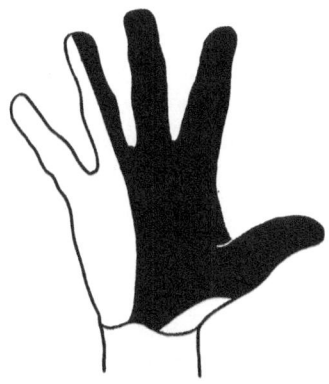

Unfortunately, symptoms can also appear in non-standard patterns, so it is not always accurate to base the diagnosis solely on the location of the symptoms. And, again, there are other conditions that can cause similar problems. That is why you need to see your PCP. But, patients with CTS often wake up with pain or numbness in the hand. If they "shake out" the hand, the symptoms temporarily resolve. In fact, that shaking out of the hand is called the "flick test" and it is both sensitive and specific for CTS.

When you see your PCP they will likely perform a couple of physical exam tests that may help with the diagnosis, or they may just refer you to an orthopedist. Nerve conduction studies are often used to confirm CTS. Nerve conduction studies test the electrical signal sent by the nerve; if there is a delay in the nerve conduction, then there is a problem with the nerve. Electromyography determines if the muscles innervated by that particular nerve have deteriorated from the nerve damage. Ultrasound can also be used to aid in the diagnosis.

If you do have CTS, the severity of your nerve entrapment will determine the appropriate treatment. In mild to moderate cases, a trial of conservative treatments is appropriate. Examples are splinting, steroid injections, physical therapy, therapeutic ultrasound, and yoga. Most patients see improvement in 2 to 6 weeks with maximum benefit at three months. However, if you have severe disease, or there is no improvement at 6 weeks, then it is time for a referral for possible surgical decompression.

I always try to use the most conservative therapy possible, but in this case it is interesting that oral steroids and NSAIDs have NOT been shown to be beneficial. Also, if the carpal tunnel is associated with pregnancy, it usually resolves after delivery.

I hope that helps. The best news is that although CTS is common, most people get relief with conservative measures, and if you do end up needing surgery, decompression provides a lasting and positive outcome in 70% to 90% of cases.

Chapter 35

LOWER LEG SWELLING

Dear Dr. Anne, my doctor keeps telling me that I need to wear compression socks, but they are so hard to put on. I truly hate them! Why can't I just take an extra water pill? Signed C, from Independence

Dear C, you are right that prescription compression socks are VERY hard to put on. But, let's discuss why your doctor wants you to wear them.

Swelling of the lower legs is extremely common as we age. It can be caused by many things, but is usually caused by a combination of a little bit of several things; sedentary life style, leaky valves in the veins of the legs (also called venous insufficiency), poor muscle tone, obesity, poor lymphatic drainage from the legs, heart disease, lung disease, kidney disease, liver disease, and more. The swelling, or edema, will not kill you, but it can cause chronic ulcers on your lower legs. The ulcers happen because skin just can't handle the constant pressure and it finally starts to break down. Once those ulcers form, it is very difficult to get them to heal because the circulation in the lower legs is so poor.

In the hospital, we don't always worry about swelling, because swelling can be a common side effect of a serious acute illness. But when it's a chronic condition, it is great that your doctor is paying attention to it. Aside from treating the cause of the swelling, which is too broad to discuss here, let's just discuss what to do about the swelling and your suggestion to take more of your water pills.

Whenever there is swelling of the lower legs, we have two choices on how to treat it. We can treat the edema mechanically, or chemically. Chemically treating the edema is taking a stronger dose of diuretic (or water pill).

By mechanically, I mean we can elevate the lower legs, we can wrap the lower legs with ACE-bandages, we can put on TED hose or compression socks. We could also have you stand up and raise up and down on your toes several hundred times, so that your muscles do the same thing as the socks. Actually, walking three miles every day would be my first choice, and that might even be enough to totally resolve your health concerns. But, with any of those options, we are trying to push the fluid out of the tissues, back into the vessels, and get it up to the kidneys. Once that happens, the kidneys will make urine out of all that fluid and you can pee it out.

In the picture below, can you see how the valves of the veins are not closing in the picture labeled venous insufficiency? When this happens, the blood pools in the lower legs and the pressure builds up in the veins. Then the liquid portion of the blood (the plasma) leaks out into the tissues causing pitting swelling.

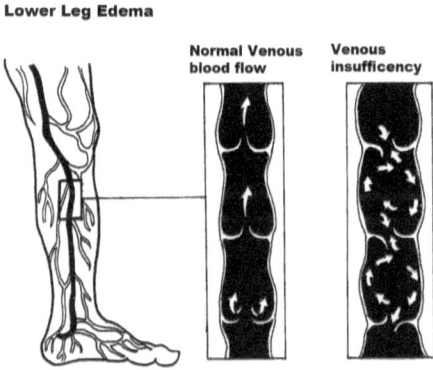

Lower Leg Edema

The pictures below show why toes raises are so important. The tensing and relaxing of the calf muscles helps "pump" the fluid up to the kidneys. The muscles can act similarly to the valves when our valves have weakened or become leaky with age. Good muscle tone and regular flexing of the calf muscles can help a great deal.

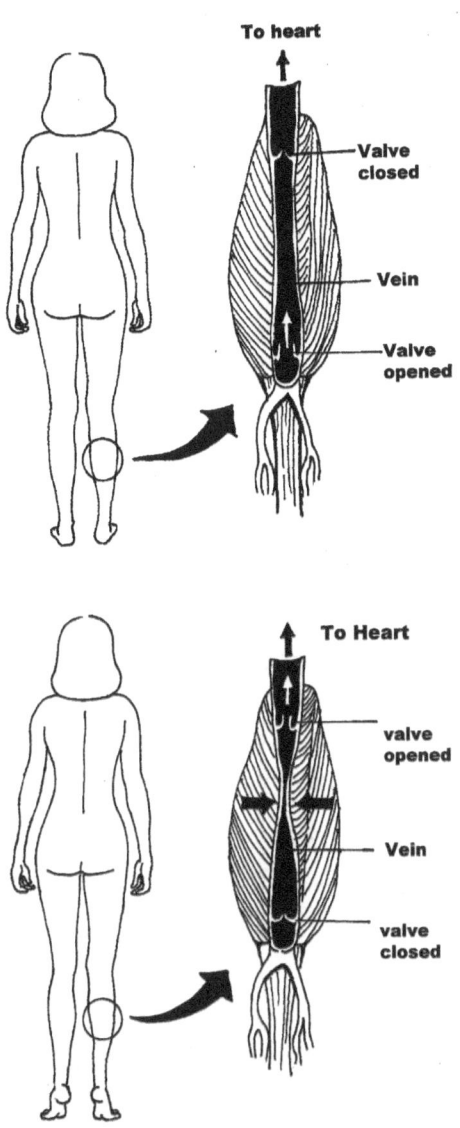

Obviously, you can't do several hundred toe raises at a time. But, if you would commit to doing 10 toe raises during every commercial break while you are watching your nightly TV, it will make an enormous difference to your overall vein health. Toe raises are shown below. Please note that I would prefer that you hold onto something for balance.

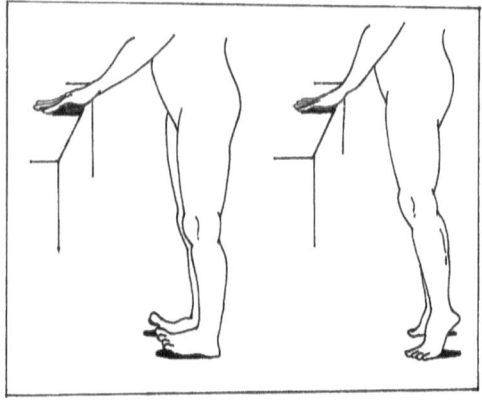

Finally, once you get the swelling down with the prescription compression socks, you may be able to change to an over-the-counter, mild compression sock. These are much easier to put on and are available from Dr. Scholl's and others, at many local drugstores, or at Walmart. You can also find them online.

Finally, there are many devices available to help you get the compression socks on, one example is shown below.

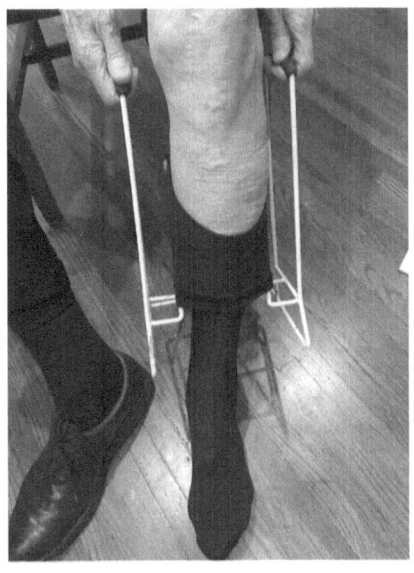

Now let's get back to your question regarding chemically treating your swelling. You are right that taking an extra water pill is much easier than getting your compression socks on. But the two strategies are not even remotely comparable. Water pills basically force your kidneys to work much harder, but they really do nothing for your lower legs. Believe me, you don't want to hammer on your kidneys; those little beans can only take so much abuse. In certain chronic disease states, we may tell the patient to take an extra water pill for three days, if their weight goes up 5 pounds. But even in that situation, they should already be wearing compression socks, or doing some other form of mechanical treatment for their edema.

My good friend, Dr. Amanda Valliant, is an interventional nephrologist (which means she is a very specialized kidney doctor) and her daily battle cry is, "Always take care of the beans!" That means take care of your kidneys! Over using your water pill will eventually just overwork your kidneys.

Chapter 36

NEW DIAGNOSIS OF DIABETES

Dear Dr. Anne, I was just diagnosed with Type II Diabetes. But, my doctor also started me on a blood pressure medication and a cholesterol medication. Why? I don't have high blood pressure and my cholesterol is a little high, but not terrible, so why do I need all these other meds? And, more importantly, is there any way to get rid of diabetes? And, why is he saying that I have to see the eye doctor and the foot doctor? I am made of questions right now! Signed R, from Coffeyville.

Dear R, darn-it, a new diagnosis of diabetes is a tough way to ring in the New Year. I love your comment about "being made of questions," and I don't blame you.

We used to think that diabetes was just high blood sugar (also called blood glucose or just glucose) and that it was no big deal. Unfortunately, we now know that diabetes is a HUGE deal and it affects essentially the whole body.

Many people know that diabetics can go into a coma and die if their blood sugar gets too low (if you're not diabetic, low blood sugars will not cause coma and death). But, many don't realize that ANY TIME the blood sugar is ABOVE normal, it damages your blood vessels, your kidneys, your eyes, and the nerves of your feet and hands, as well as the nerves that control your intestines. That is why most diabetics die of coronary artery disease. And, this is why diabetes is the leading cause of end stage kidney disease, which means that the patient has to be on dialysis, or they will die. And, this is why diabetics can go blind. And, why so many diabetics have neuropathy, meaning that they have constant burning or numbness in their feet and sometimes hands.

When someone has a new diagnosis of Type II diabetes, first and foremost, your doctor should talk to you about changing the way you eat and exercising more. After diet and exercise, every new Type II diabetic should be started on a medication called Metformin. This medication slows down of the effect of what you've eaten on your blood sugar. That is kind of hard to explain; let me try again. Metformin slows down how quickly the sugar in the food you have eaten is released into the blood stream. It also seems to give some protection to the heart.

However, there are a couple of problems with Metformin. The first issue is that it tends to cause GI upset and diarrhea. Usually, this subsides in a few days, but not always. Most doctors will start you at 500 mg with breakfast for a week, and make sure that at the end of the week you are not having any GI upset. The second week you will take 500 mg with breakfast and 500 mg with your evening meal. The third week you would take 1000 mg with breakfast and 500 mg with the evening meal, and the fourth week you would take 1000 mg twice daily with meals. If at any time you cannot get over the GI upset then you would either go back down to the previous dose, or there is a long acting form of Metformin, that is more expensive, and you could try that. Most people get used to Metformin, but not everyone can tolerate it. In addition, if you have a significant amount of kidney dysfunction, then Metformin is contraindicated (cannot be taken).

Now, Metformin alone may not be enough to control your blood sugar, but that is where we usually start. After that, there are many other drugs to try but I won't go into all those options here. That is another huge topic.

Recall that I said that diabetes affects the whole body, so we can't worry about the blood sugar alone. We have to start trying to protect the kidneys, the vessels, the heart, etc. To protect the kidneys we need to start a medication in the class called ACE-Inhibitors. All the ACE-Inhibitors end in "pril." Examples are Lisinopril, Benazepril, Enalapril, Captopril, and Ramipril, but the list goes on. They are all about the same effectiveness and Lisinopril is almost always the cheapest. What is so interesting is that these medications were developed to control blood pressure, but we have found that they help protect the kidneys from diabetes and they help the heart in congestive heart failure. So, even if your blood pressure is fine, your doctor will likely start you on a small dose of Lisinopril or another of the ACE-Inhibitors. Patients with high blood pressure may need 40 mg of Lisinopril daily. A patient without hypertension, but with diabetes, would still benefit from 2.5 or 5 mg of Lisinopril daily.

The next most important thing is to protect your vessels and in particular, the vessels of your heart. We know that diabetes is pro-atherosclerotic. That means that diabetes itself causes plaques in the vessels. When a plaque in a vessel ruptures, the gooey stuff inside spills out and clogs the vessel downstream. If that vessel is providing blood to the heart, then you have a myocardial infarction (also called an MI, which a lot of people call a heart attack). Diabetes is considered a "cardiovascular equivalent." That means that it is just as much of a risk factor for MI as having had a previous MI. In other words, it is the same risk as having KNOWN coronary artery disease.

"Statins" are the best medication to keep those plaques stable, so they won't rupture. Examples of "Statins" are simvastatin, lovastatin, pravastatin, atorvastatin, and of course there are more, but they all end in "statin." These drugs do lower your cholesterol, but more importantly, they stabilize the plaques that are forming just because you have diabetes.

Yipes! This column is already too long, so I have to stop. But, actually, I am thrilled that your doctor is so thorough. I assume that he/she has started you on Metformin, Lisinopril (or another ACE-Inhibitor) and Simvastatin (or another Statin) and if so, I would say he or she is doing things just right. Let's talk more about your other questions next week.

Chapter 37

NEW DIABETES, PART 2

For anyone who might have missed my column two weeks ago, "R" is a newly diagnosed type II diabetic and he/she had several questions about this very important and all-encompassing disease. Two weeks ago I tried to answer R's question about why his/her doctor had prescribed other medications beside blood sugar meds. Today, I am going to try to answer R's second question, which was, "Is there any way to get rid of diabetes?"

First, I need to make sure that we are all talking about the same disease state. This column is about **Type II Diabetes Mellitus**, this is **NOT** about Type I Diabetes Mellitus, and it is **NOT** about Diabetes Insipidus.

But, to answer your question, **YES** type II diabetes mellitus, is sometimes curable. Of course this is qualified and we don't understand all of it, but here is what we know. There are two ways to "cure" diabetes.

First, Roux-en-Y bariatric surgeries cure diabetes. We don't really understand why this is true, but we just know that in most cases, the patient is no longer diabetic when they leave the hospital after surgery. On occasion, it may take closer to a week. But, the patient is usually cured of their diabetes even BEFORE the weight loss happens. AND, they will remain cured as long as their BMI remains within the normal range. The problem is that surgery is expensive, painful, and dangerous. And, it is important to point out that even though the diabetes was cured before the weight loss happened, if the weight comes back, they will likely become diabetic again. Again, I don't understand that, I just know that it is true.

The only other way to "cure" diabetes is to dramatically reduce your insulin needs. To understand this, we have to understand insulin a little better.

If you recall from last week, I said that anytime the blood sugar is higher than normal, it is damaging your organs. Therefore, when the blood sugar is high, the pancreas is stimulated to secrete more insulin. The insulin opens the "door" (actually called a receptor) to the fat cells to allow the sugar to leave the blood stream and enter the fat cells. Once inside the fat cells, the sugar is converted into more fat.

Insulin can also open the door to the muscle cells to allow sugar to enter the muscle, but only if the muscle is calling for more sugar at that time. The only way for that to happen is if you happen to be exercising that muscle really hard at the time that your blood sugar is high. I don't know about you, but when my blood sugar is high it is usually when I am pushing back from the table saying, "Why did I eat that?" I can't think of a single time when I was eating cheesecake while running really hard.

Anyway, the vast majority of the time, insulin doesn't open the receptor on the muscle cells, instead it opens the glucose receptor on the fat cells. And once inside the fat cell, the sugar or glucose is converted into more fat. In type II diabetes, the blood sugar has been chronically high, and the pancreas has been making more and more insulin to try to deal with the high blood sugars. Finally, the fat cells stop responding to the insulin. Even though the insulin has attached to the receptor to open it, the receptor won't open. This is called "insulin resistance."

Once the patient is insulin resistant, the changes really have to be dramatic. Simple carbohydrates ALWAYS increase blood sugar and therefore ALWAYS increase insulin needs. Proteins and fats do NOT increase blood sugar and do NOT increase insulin needs. We know that even after insulin resistance sets in, a dramatic decrease in the consumption of carbohydrates will start to "wake up" the fat cells. If the very low carbohydrate diet is maintained, the fat cells will again have a normal response to insulin when it is occasionally increased to deal with a high blood sugar level.

I know that these are both dramatic changes. The truth is that the body is incredibly complex and we just don't understand all of it. Type II diabetes is a breakdown in the body's ability to maintain balance. It is a result of chronic misuse. The body is not meant to handle daily doses of sugar and other simple carbohydrates. The body is meant to consume meat, eggs, vegetables, fruits, nuts and dairy, with a few simple carbs thrown in.

After all, what is a Funyun, anyway? What are cheese doodles? What are Ramen Noodles? What are Cocoa Puffs made of and why in the world do we give them to our children – the greatest treasure God has gifted us with? I know they taste good and are cheap, but these things have no nutritional value and in fact are detrimental. Eaten occasionally, our bodies are wonderfully designed to handle them. Eaten daily, these things constantly flood our systems with sugar and our bodies just can't deal with it.

So, R, the answer to your question, is yes, diabetes can sometimes be defeated. But, you are going to have to make major changes in your life to back out of this terrible disease.

Chapter 38

SHOULD I BE TAKING ASPIRIN DAILY?

Dear Dr. Anne, I am 59 years old and I am trying to decide whether to take a daily baby aspirin or not. Some say yes, and some say no. What do you say? Signed E from Independence.

Dear E, yours is an excellent question, and mine will, unfortunately, be a confusing answer. First, it is confusing because the guidelines have changed, and second, it is confusing because the answer is no longer universal.

Let me explain.

As recently as 2011, it was recommended that everyone over the age of 50 take a baby aspirin (81 mg) every day as a preventative measure. The reasoning was that platelets are involved in clot and plaque formation, and aspirin is an anti-platelet drug, so we knew that a small daily dose of aspirin would reduce blood clots and plaques, which can contribute to ischemic strokes, heart attacks, and other vessel problems that become a common problem as we age.

However, as we have continued to study preventative medicine, we now separate "primary" and "secondary" prevention. "Primary Prevention" means that you are doing something, or taking something, that will help you to avoid ever having a particular event or a disease (like a heart attack, or a stroke, or a cancer). "Secondary Prevention" means that you are doing something, or taking something, that will help you not have ANOTHER event, like a second stroke or a second heart attack.

Also remember, EVERY drug you take has side effects. I'll say it another way. There is NO such things as a drug completely free of side effects. The key is to determine whether the benefits outweigh the risks. With aspirin, as is true with **ANY** NSAID (aspirin, ibuprofen, naproxen, meloxicam, diclofenac, etc.) the risks are:
  1) bleeding – usually in the form of peptic ulcer disease, but the bleeding can be anywhere,
  2) worsening heart failure, and
  3) worsening kidney disease.

So if you are already dealing with **ANY** of those three issues, the risks likely outweigh the benefits and you should probably NOT take a baby aspirin daily.

So, what are the benefits of a daily baby aspirin?

For "Primary Prevention" of heart attack and stroke, the USPSTF (US Preventative Services Task Force) currently recommends that doctors tell their patients:
  1) Aspirin is recommended for men ages 45 to 79 to reduce the risk of **heart attack** *when a net benefit is present.*
  2) Aspirin is recommended for women ages 55 to 79 to reduce the risk of **ischemic stroke** *when a net benefit is present.*

Why only until age 79? Well after that age, the risk of bleed increases, which changes the risk/benefit ratio making the risks likely higher than the benefits. The second question is, "What do they mean, '*when is there a net benefit?*'"

A net benefit is present when there is a moderate to high risk for heart attack or ischemic stroke. For men, the risk factors for heart attack are:

1) Hypertension - is your blood pressure high OR are you taking medications to keep it within the normal limits?
2) Is your total cholesterol level high or is your "LDL cholesterol, also called bad cholesterol" level high and your "HDL cholesterol, also called good cholesterol" level low?
3) Do you have diabetes?
4) Are you a smoker?

If you are male, between 45 and 79 years old, and any of those apply to you, *then a daily baby aspirin would provide a net benefit to you*, which means it has been shown to reduce your risk of heart attack.

For women, the risks of ischemic stroke are:

1) Hypertension - is your blood pressure high OR are you taking medications to keep it within the normal limits?
2) Do you have thickening (hypertrophy) of the heart walls due to high blood pressure?
3) Do you have diabetes?
4) Do you have coronary artery disease? Have you had a previous stent, or coronary artery bypass surgery?
5) Are you a smoker?

If you are female, between the ages of 55 and 79, and any of those apply to you, *then a daily baby aspirin would provide a net benefit to you*, which means it has been shown to reduce your risk of ischemic stroke.

Another factor to consider regarding "Primary Prevention" is that a 2012 review in the journal "Lancet Oncology" found that taking a daily baby aspirin may reduce your risk of certain types of cancer. I know that is a bit nebulous, but it is too long a subject to go into now.

A daily baby aspirin gives "Secondary Prevention" in the following cases:

1) If you have coronary artery disease, meaning you have had either a stent placed, or have had a coronary artery bypass graft, then a daily baby aspirin has been shown to reduce the occurrence of further coronary artery blockages.

2) If you have had stents placed in other places besides the heart, like your legs or your neck, then a daily baby aspirin has been shown to reduce the occurrence of additional blockages.

3) If you have had a stroke or a TIA (transient ischemic attack – also called a "mini stroke") then a baby aspirin every day has been shown to reduce the occurrence of additional TIA's or a second stroke.

So, I can see why you were confused. Heck, I get confused and I study medicine every day! It is truly NOT the clear cut answer that we used to think it was. But, please don't get frustrated. Medicine keeps changing because our bodies are incredibly complex and we are constantly trying to do a better job of understanding them. I am just glad that you asked, because it means that you are engaged and paying attention to your health. That is the most important part of maintaining a good quality of life. So, thanks for asking!

Chapter 39

THE VITAMIN D DEFICIENCY CONUNDRUM

Dear Dr. Anne, at my last physical, my physician ordered blood work that included checking for Vitamin D. My Vitamin D level was 21, which prompted my physician to prescribe over-the-counter Vitamin D3 supplements. As I researched on the internet, it seems low Vitamin D is a common condition. Since Vitamin D is so important for bodily functions, why don't basic blood panels include a test for it? Thanks, L from Independence.

Dear L, thank you for your excellent question; I would love to talk about Vitamin D.

There is no escaping the fact that we humans get most of our Vitamin D from the conversion of sunlight to the active form of Vitamin D in our bodies. Back in the old days, when people spent more time outdoors, and sunscreen was unheard of, Vitamin D deficiencies were practically non-existent. But it is hard to balance our need for Vitamin D with the fact that skin cancer, from sun exposure, is an equally huge problem in our population.

We can get Vitamin D from some foods, but very few foods naturally contain Vitamin D. Fish livers are the biggest source of Vitamin D, and although I am happy to eat fish a couple of times a week, I am not keen on eating the liver of said fish! Luckily, many of our foods have supplemental Vitamin D added.

The answer to your question is that most doctors don't routinely test for Vitamin D Deficiency, because most insurance won't cover it. The only cases that I know of where insurance will cover the cost to test the Vitamin D level in the blood is if you have one of the following:

1) a recent fracture,
2) some condition that causes malabsorption (meaning that you cannot absorb the vitamin D that is in your food or in your supplements – this usually happens if you have had bariatric surgery, or you have celiac, or Crohn's, or pancreatic insufficiency, or cystic fibrosis, etc.), or
3) you have a condition that keeps you from converting the sunlight absorbed by the skin into the active form of Vitamin D that your body can use. This can happen with either chronic kidney disease or chronic liver disease.

Vitamin D is extremely important, and deficiencies of Vitamin D are now very common, so YES I would love it if we routinely checked Vitamin D levels in everyone. Since your insurance won't cover it, in my mind, the answer is that everyone should be taking daily vitamin D supplements. The current standard recommendations are that EVERYONE between the ages of 1 and 70 needs 600 international units of Vitamin D daily. And, that EVERYONE over the age of 70 needs 800 international units of Vitamin D daily.

Vitamin D is cheap and in the quantity listed above it is completely safe. BUT, remember that it is a fat soluble vitamin which means that it can build up in your system. Although rare, Vitamin D toxicity is not unheard of, so don't overdo. Some doctors will prescribe high dose Vitamin D once weekly for a short period of time in those that are deficient, but this practice has become controversial. That is why most physicians just recommend that everyone take the daily supplement that I listed above.

Chapter 40

VITAMIN D VS SKIN CANCER

Dear Dr. Anne, Last week, in your column about vitamin D you commented that vitamin D deficiencies were rare in the past and are common now -- because we don't get in the sun. And, of course we don't get in the sun because YOU TOLD US NOT TO! So what exactly are you recommending? Thanks, M, from Independence.

Dear M, Yikes, I can see what you mean about my recommendations not being clear. In my defense, this question requires a juggling act, but let me see if I can do a better job.

First, let me make it clear that our bodies are designed to make the vitamin D that we need from sunlight. Sixty years ago, central air conditioning, 300 channels of television, computer solitaire, and Candy Crush were not available. We, as a society, spent a lot more time outside than we do today.

Skin cancer was not a huge concern 60 years ago. First, we just didn't know as much about it then. But, secondly, we weren't living as long as we are now, so skin cancers didn't have time to become such a problem. It takes years for skin cancers (other than melanomas) to become an issue. In 1950, the average U.S. life span was about 67 years. Today, the average U.S. life span is more like 80 years. Ten tiny squamous cell carcinomas might not even be noticed at age 67. But, at age 80, those same small cancers have become a much bigger problem.

I would like to mention one more thing about life span that seems to be developing in our area. If you read the local obituaries, you may have noticed that there seems to be a "bi-modal" pattern to lifespans. By that I mean that there are an awful lot of people that are passing in their 50's and early 60's, and then another group that is passing much later, in their 80's and 90's and every once in a while, even 100's. And, although I have not found studies that give explicit data on this, it often seems to be related to lifestyle choices.

I have taken care of some wonderful people who passed at a young age because they were unlucky enough to be dealing with a particularly aggressive cancer, but that is not the norm. Much more often those loved ones that we are losing early, have been struggling with uncontrolled diabetes, uncontrolled hypertension, regular use of cocaine or methamphetamines, heavy alcohol use, or heavy tobacco use; in other words, lifestyle choices.

I appreciate that you are holding me accountable on being clear in my recommendations. But, my real recommendation is that there is absolutely no substitute for the basics.

1) Exercise regularly. It is not enough just to stay busy. Your body needs regular exercise. If your joints or your back won't let you walk or jog, then get in the pool and swim laps or do water aerobics, or dance, or lift weights.

2) Stay away from junk food. Eat only food that your body will benefit from. Many items that we call "food" have no nutritional value at all, so they really shouldn't even be called food. We all tend to think that if someone is thin, they can eat whatever they want. But, that is just not the case. Unhealthy food is STILL unhealthy, no matter what you weigh.

3) Maintain a healthy weight. I have talked about this one many times and it is true that it is much more difficult

than it was 60 years ago. Servings are larger for everything and sugar is added to almost everything. But, just because it is harder, doesn't mean that we don't have to do it.

4) Find a way to deal with the stress in your life. Whether it is prayer, or meditation, or exercise, or a hobby, or a regular massage; I don't care what you choose. The fact is that any pain is worse when there is also depression or stress. And, depression and stress are worse when there is pain. It becomes a terrible cycle.

5) Stop smoking, or at least cut down to less than 10 cigarettes a day. Drink alcohol only moderately – multiple drinks daily is too much for your liver. Just because Sherlock Holmes used cocaine does not mean that you should; he was fictional, you and I are not. Cocaine and meth will kill you, period.

Did this just become a rant? I'm sorry, I really do apologize. It is just so hard to see people dying 30 years earlier than they should.

Chapter 41

DIET COMPARISON

Dear Dr. Anne, my doctor has told me that the reason my back and knees and ankles hurt so much is that I am too heavy. I can't stand this pain, so I know I have to make a change. But, how do I decide what diet plan is best? Do you recommend Weight Watchers, the Paleo Diet, or the Low-Carb Diet? Signed T, from Independence.

Dear T, Congratulations! I am so glad that you have made the decision to make a change! That is the first step and it is a big one.

I would like to encourage you to make a distinction in your own mind here at the beginning. Please try not to think of this as "going on a diet." That phrase implies that this is a temporary change and once you have lost weight, you will go back to your previous eating habits. Instead, try to think of this as a life-style change. You are starting a new chapter and you are going to be stronger, more energetic, and have less pain, and most importantly, you will continue on in your new healthy state *FOR LIFE.*

As you said, the next step is deciding how to go about this new chapter. There are lots of ways to lose weight and improve how you feel. All three plans that you mentioned have worked for many people, the most important thing is to find out what works for you. But, there are of course pros and cons to every diet plan.

Weight Watchers

The thing that I love about Weight Watchers is that you are part of a group with an inherent support system. As long as you continue to go to the meetings, you have someone to encourage you and keep you on track and that is HUGE. What I don't like about Weight Watchers is something I hear from some attendees (although this might not be what the leaders are actually saying). That is that they can still have the same foods that they have eaten before, but they just need to eat them in smaller quantities. This bothers me for two reasons, (1) unhealthy foods are still unhealthy, and (2) if you and I had the discipline to stop eating with a very small portion, then we wouldn't be having this discussion in the first place.

I am not saying that you can never have a splurge, but if I can have French fries, or pasta, or rice, or mashed potatoes, or ice cream, but I can only have ¼-½ cup of it, that is just going to make me crazy. Even if I get through that first meal without diving into a larger portion, every time I open the fridge and see the container of linguini there, that I am not allowed to have until tomorrow, I am going to be really hard to get along with. First because it is going to take all of my focus just to stay out of the dang pasta, but also because eating those simple carbs daily, EVEN in small quantities, sends my blood sugar on a terrible roller coaster and makes me crave those simple carbs even more. So, for those reasons, Weight Watcher's is not a great option for me.

Paleo Diet

For those who may not have heard of this diet, the goal is to eat like humans did back when we were in the "hunter/gatherer" stage. So, unprocessed meats, vegetables, fruits, nuts and seeds are the staples of the Paleo Diet. It should include lots of raw and organic foods and no processed foods. That means no dairy, and no grains, which means no flour, so obviously no bread (which means no crackers, no bagels, no tortillas), no oats, no rice, no pasta, no cereal, etc. It does allow honey and maple syrup.

My concern with the Paleo Diet is that, (1) it would be too easy for me to screw it up, and (2) I don't think I would ever feel satisfied.

For example, honey and maple syrup are natural, but they are still sugar and they have the same effect on your blood glucose that sugar does. When we were hunter/gatherers we couldn't go buy a jar of honey and drizzle it over anything that lacked flavor, but I certainly can – and I am afraid that I would.

Nuts are another problem for me. I love them and it is darn hard to be reasonable in how much I eat. I need to be able to feel that I am not denying myself. I can walk away from a piece of pie if I have been satisfied with roasted pork, and melted cheddar cheese rolled up in a low carb tortilla. But, I don't know that I could if I had had a grilled chicken breast with a side of eggplant and water cress; which leads me to the Low-Carb diet.

Low-Carb Diet

The Low-Carb Diet still has millions of variations, but that just means that you can continue to tailor it to your needs. In general, every time you eat you need to eat more grams of protein than "net carbs" and try to keep your total net carb in take less than or equal to 30 grams in a 24 hours period. People calculate "net carbs" in 2 different ways.

Net Carbs (g) = Total Carbohydrates (g) – Dietary Fiber (g)

Or the more lenient calculation is:

Net Carbs (g) = Total Carbohydrates (g) - [Dietary Fiber (g) + ½ Sugar Alcohols (g)]

(Except if that sugar alcohol is Erythritol, which is a sugar alcohol with a glycemic index of zero – so it has no impact on your blood sugar. Then you don't have to include it in your calculation.)

Again, no matter which way you calculate your "net carbs," you should keep your total "net carb" intake below 30 grams per day.

I prefer this diet because if I want eggs and bacon and a bit of fruit for breakfast, I can have them. I just can't have toast and hash browns with it. If I want a big juicy steak for dinner, I can have it with a big salad or sautéed veggies. I just can't have fries, or a big baked potato with it. And the great thing about this diet is that it dramatically lowers your insulin needs. In our society, where diabetes is rampant, this is a huge benefit.

I have hit my word limit on words for this column and I need to stop writing, but let me end by suggesting some books that are easy to read and VERY inspiring.

"The New Atkins for the New You"

"Why We Get Fat and What to do about it"

"Wheat Belly"

"Taking Out the Carbage"

Again, please let me congratulate you on your decision. No matter how you go about it, you are going to feel so much better!

Chapter 42

WEIGHT LOSS AT THE END OF LIFE

Dear Dr. Anne, my Mom is on hospice and she is getting terribly thin, she just looks awful. I asked the hospice nurse what we can do about it and she had no recommendations. I know that I have heard of appetite stimulators in the past. Why isn't someone giving her something? Signed N, from Independence.

Dear N, I am so sorry about your Mom. I know it is hard to watch and you feel helpless, while she seems to be wasting away before your eyes. But, let me share the most current recommendations with you, which I hope will give you some peace.

Weight loss is almost universally a part of the final phase of most terminal diseases. This weight loss is called "cachexia" by doctors and nurses and it is defined as the severe loss of both muscle and fat when the patient is not trying to lose weight.

Cachexia is caused by complex changes in the body during the last chapter of life. It starts with changes in the nervous system, which alters the hormone regulation of the body, which, in turn, affects the metabolism of the body. As a result, the patient's appetite is suppressed, and the body starts burning more muscle, which of course causes more weight loss.

As you mentioned, we used to treat this with appetite stimulators like dronabinol, megestrol, medical marijuana, and others. Unfortunately, only 20 to 30% of the patients who take these drugs gain any weight at all. And, more importantly, for those patients who are able to gain weight, studies have shown that there is no improvement in quality of life or in mortality.

Doctors have also tried feeding these patients in every way imaginable. We have fed them intravenously, through a nasogastric tube (a tube entering the nose and going into the stomach), through a nasojejunal tube (a tube entering the nose and going down to the jejunum –past the stomach into the second part of the small intestine), and even through a percutaneous endoscopic gastrostomy tube (PEG tube – where liquid nutrition is given directly into the stomach), and none of these interventions have reversed the weight loss, or improved either quality of life or mortality. Moreover, they all have associated risk and discomfort; every patient that I have ever treated, who had an NG tube in their nose, was very anxious to get it out! As a result of these failed attempts, newer definitions of cachexia often read, "weight loss that cannot be reversed with increased calorie consumption."

So, I am sorry, but I don't have an easy answer for you. If your Mom is hungry, she should eat, but there is no benefit to encouraging her to eat. I often hear families say to their loved one, who is a hospice patient, "You have to eat and keep your strength up," and I know they are just expressing their love and concern. But in fact, the patient should to do whatever makes them most comfortable. Once the patient is being treated by a hospice group, comfort is all that matters. I know it is easy for me to say this, and very hard to do, but try to be at peace with her weight loss. It is an inevitable part of the journey.

Chapter 43

WHAT ABOUT MEDS FOR OSTEOPOROSIS?

Dear Dr. Anne, I recently got a bone scan that said that I have osteoporosis. I have done a lot of investigation online that says that if I take calcium and exercise, I should not have to take prescription medicine for my bones. Please tell me that what I have read is correct! Signed, K from Independence.

Dear K, I love that you are involved in your health and interested in investigating all options. But, PLEASE take the prescription meds on this one. Let me explain.

You may already know this, but for those readers who don't, osteoporosis is a condition where the bones become weak. That means you are at increased risk for fractures, usually hip and wrist fractures from a fall that would normally not break a bone. You probably also know that it is incredibly common for elderly patients to fracture a hip, and make it through the surgery to fix the fracture, but then pass away either in the post op period or in the 4 months following surgery due to pneumonia or a myriad of other complications. Suffice it to say that although hip fractures are common, they greatly increase the mortality of that patient and are a really big deal in the world of geriatric medicine.

However, they are not what scare me the most about osteoporosis. What really scares me is the increased risk of vertebral fractures. When a vertebra is fractured it is called a compression fracture. Do you see in the diagram below how the fractured vertebrae are shorter than the others? And, notice that the nerves that exit the spine at that point are being compressed also. Compressed nerves cause pain and lots of it! There will be incredible pain not only in the back and but also in whatever distribution that nerve supplies.

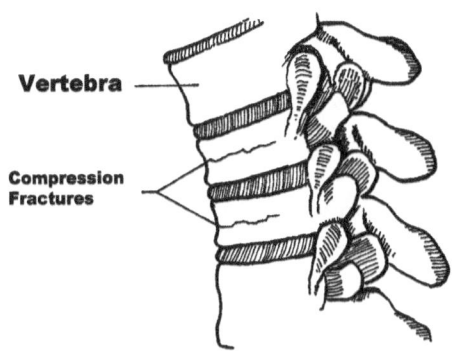

Vertebra

Compression Fractures

We can sometimes treat compression fractures with a process called kyphoplasty, where a "cement" is injected into the crushed bone to restore the previous architecture and relieve the pressure on the nerve – see the illustration below.

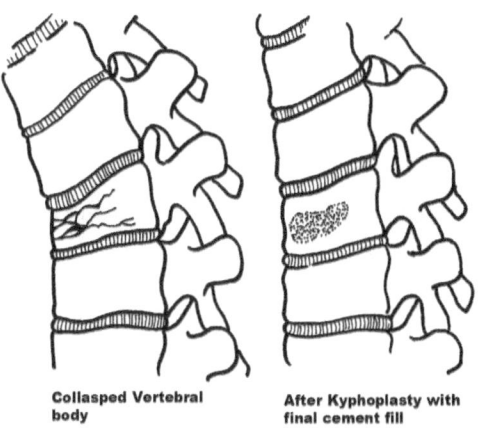

Collasped Vertebral body

After Kyphoplasty with final cement fill

I love that we can do this, and usually things work out great. But, it just doesn't always work. Unfortunately, I have treated patients where the kyphoplasty didn't work and they are left in constant and unremitting pain. I think I could probably handle a lot in life, but relentless pain is one thing that I really would like to avoid.

Although I take a calcium supplement daily and recommend that most other women do too, studies have not shown that calcium supplementation actually reduces the incidence of fractures. So, why do I take them? Well, I notice a difference in my fingernails when I stop taking calcium. So, whether supported by medical evidence or not, I figure it is supplying something that I am not getting in my diet.

I guess my question to you is, "Why are you not wanting to take the medication?" There are lots of options for these meds; some are taken orally, some are injected once a month, others once every 6 months and others once yearly. Really, compared to dying my hair every month, these meds are not really that big an ordeal.

The most common side effect of the most common med for osteoporosis (alendronate) is heartburn, and if that happens you should not use it anymore, and instead use one of the other drugs. There is a very rare, but terrifying side effect of alendronate – necrosis of the jaw – where the jaw bone starts dying. There is no doubt that necrosis of the jaw sounds unspeakably horrible, but not only have I never seen it, I have not even heard of another doctor that has ever seen it. So, it is pretty rare.

K, you didn't share your age or how bad your osteoporosis is, or what other risk factors you have for fractures, but if I were in your shoes, I would take the meds.

Chapter 44

THE SLEEP CONUNDRUM

Dear Dr. Anne, I have been taking Ambien every night for a long time and sleeping well. Now my doctor doesn't want to prescribe it for me. What is the big deal with Ambien? I can't sleep well without it. Signed, H from Independence.

Dear H, I too have had patients who were very upset with me because I wouldn't continually prescribe Ambien. Unfortunately, because of its many adverse side effects, Ambien is only approved for short term use AND it is only approved for a max of 10 mg in men and 5 mg in women.

Common side effects include memory loss, loss of coordination, headache, muscle pain, nausea, constipation, diarrhea, upset stomach, daytime drowsiness, dizziness, weakness, light headedness, dry mouth, nose and throat irritation, stuffy nose, and feeling "drugged." Also, Ambien is very addictive and many people really struggle to get off of it.

But the most concerning side effect of Ambien is referred to as "Ambien blackouts." The original information on Ambien listed sleep walking, abnormal thinking, and strange behavior as rare side effects. However, "sleep eating," "sleep driving," and "sleep shopping," have all been repeatedly reported. People have been in car accidents as a result of "sleep driving" while on Ambien. Ambien was even implicated in a murder trial in 2009. A friend of mine had gotten to the point where she couldn't sleep without taking Ambien, but she would occasionally wake up in someone else's home when she did take it – it was terrifying.

Good sleep can be tough especially as we age. We would all like to have that wonderful restful 8 hours of sleep that we had when we were young, but the fact is that sometimes we just can't get to sleep or can't stay asleep, even when we are mentally exhausted. If you are like me, there are about 2 nights a week where I just can't get to sleep. Medicating a two-night-a-week sleep initiation problem is not appropriate – eventually, our bodies will get tired enough that we will fall asleep.

For those nights that we all have when we just can't sleep, try not to let yourself get frustrated. If you start the, "WHY CAN'T I GET TO SLEEP?" question, your frustration and agitation will just escalate and any opportunity for rest really deteriorates. Try keeping a really boring book handy for those nights. Don't pick up an exciting spy novel, but a text book will often help you nod off.

Melatonin is an over the counter medication that is generally considered very safe and effective. I definitely recommend it. If you are over 65, please do not get started using Benadryl (also called diphenhydramine) or anything with diphenhydramine in it, like Tylenol PM. Diphenhydramine is a strong anticholinergic, which I can't go into here, but it should not be used frequently in the elderly.

But, what should you do if you are having trouble sleeping EVERY night? First, if you are having trouble staying asleep, or if you snore, or wake up with a headache, or wake up not feeling rested, or fall asleep during the day when you don't want to, then you probably need to be evaluated for Obstructive Sleep Apnea (OSA), which we talked about in an earlier column. Assuming that you do not have OSA, Sleep Doctors talk a lot about "Sleep Hygiene" which involves the following:

1) Going to bed at the same time every night and getting up at the same time every morning

2) Having a routine prior to going to bed – something like, dinner at 6 pm, evening activities until 9:30 pm, shower, and be in bed by 10 pm

3) Use your bed only for sleeping and making love – absolutely no reading in bed or watching TV in bed

4) No strenuous exercise after dinner that will increase your heart rate and your metabolism, but definitely get some sort of strenuous exercise earlier in the day (your muscles need to be tired)

5) Avoid alcohol and nicotine in the evenings

6) Avoid all sources of caffeine – unfortunately, that includes chocolate – remember, caffeine has a 25 hour half-life (that means ½ of the caffeine that you consumed will be out of your system in 25 hours)

7) No napping during the day

8) Keep the bedroom dark at night

If those things don't help, then the Sleep Doctors usually prescribe "Sleep Restriction Therapy." It works like this: say you are going to bed every night at 10 pm and lying there awake until 1 am when you finally fall asleep and sleep until 6 am. Your "Sleep Restriction Therapy" regimen would start with you getting in bed at 1 am and setting your alarm and getting up at 6 am. After several days of that, you go to bed at 12:45 am and set the alarm for 6 am. And, continue on every 5 to 7 days, giving yourself an additional 15 minutes of sleep time, until you are at a level of about 7 to 8 hours of sleep. Although, it is true that many of us never get to 8 hours regularly.

Or, if you go to bed at 10 pm and awaken every morning at 3 am then, your "Sleep Restriction Therapy" regimen would be to go to bed at 10 pm and set the alarm for 3 am. After 5 to 7 days, go to bed at 10 pm and set the alarm for 3:15 am. Then, continue on giving yourself another 15 minutes of sleep every 5 to 7 days until you are getting a reasonable amount of sleep.

Getting a good 8 hours of sleep EVERY night is just not in the cards for most adults. There are always times when the stresses of life make sleep difficult. Prayer, meditation, exercise, yoga, talking with a friend or a counselor, taking a walk in the woods, or reading poetry are all great ways to calm your mind and prepare yourself for resting. I know there are still some providers that are writing prescriptions for Ambien nightly, but most have stopped doing that because of the unpredictable and often dangerous consequences. Ambien is a reasonable option for an occasional night when you cannot sleep, but the benefits of nightly use just don't outweigh the risks and the insurance companies are starting to really frown on doctors who prescribe it nightly.

Chapter 45

THE ORBERA PROCEDURE

Dear Dr. Anne, I have struggled with my weight for years. I have recently heard about a new weight loss procedure called ORBERA. Please tell me what you think of it. Signed, C from Coffeyville.

Dear C, thanks for asking. I don't know a ton about the procedure, but I am excited by what I do know. First, let me assure you that the procedure is not new. It has been used in over eighty other countries for many years; it is just new to us in the U.S. So don't feel like you will be a guinea pig. Basically, a soft silicone balloon is placed in the stomach and then filled with saline. This inflated balloon takes up room, so you get full more quickly.

It may sound complicated but it's really not. The ORBERA balloon is placed in the stomach by a surgeon during an outpatient procedure. You are given a mild sedative and then a tube is passed down into your stomach from your mouth. The deflated silicon balloon is passed through the tube and down into the stomach. Then the balloon is filled with saline through a self-sealing valve. When the balloon is filled it is about the size of a grapefruit. The entire placement procedure takes 20 to 30 minutes and there is no cutting, stitching, stapling, etc.

While the balloon is in place it slows down the digestion of the food in your stomach, and of course, you won't feel the need to eat as much as you have in the past. Hence, you lose weight. It is not that you will never be hungry, but you will feel full much more quickly and you will get used to eating much less. At the end of a maximum of six months, the procedure is reversed. Once again, you get the mild sedative and the tube is inserted down through the esophagus into the stomach. This time the balloon is deflated and removed. Again, there's no cutting, no stitching, no scars.

From what I have read, most of the medical centers doing this procedure see the patient regularly during the 6 months while the balloon is in place, and for 6 months afterwards. These appointments are an effort to help you develop good eating habits with reasonable portion control after the balloon is removed, as well as developing and maintaining an exercise program. When you think about the fact that it really takes much less than 6 months to break the habit of overeating and to institute a new habit of portion control – you can see the reasoning behind this procedure.

The ORBERA website states that you can expect to lose up to 33 pounds during the six month process.

You might wonder how this procedure compares to bariatric surgery. The ORBERA procedure is actually targeted to patients who have a BMI of less than 35. Bariatric surgery, on the other hand, targets those with BMI greater than 35, or those with disease processes that have been caused by their excess weight.

There is no doubt that bariatric surgery works. People lose a lot of weight after bariatric surgery (typically more than from the ORBERA system) and most people (but certainly not all people) keep it off. But, depending on the type of bariatric surgery that you have, there can be some serious complications. Besides the immediate complications of the surgery itself, there can be mal-absorption problems in the years that follow. Because the ORBERA procedure is not removing any of your GI-tract malabsorption is not an issue.

From what I have seen, the cost of ORBERA ranges from a very minimum of $3,000 up to $9,000 with the vast majority somewhere in $6,000-$7,000 range. And, I have heard that this procedure will soon be offered at Wilson County Medical Center.

Of course, you still have to change your eating habits and hold onto those new healthier eating habits once the balloon has been removed. Any time that I talk to people about weight loss or exercise, I try to remind them that changes should ALWAYS be life-style changes, NOT short term fixes followed by a return to the poor habits that we had in the past. It is critical that we each evaluate why we are eating and try to eat only when we are hungry; not because we are tired, or angry, or worried, or anxious, or celebrating, or anything else.

Chapter 46

WHAT ABOUT MY THIGH PAIN?

Dear Dr. Anne, I'm really struggling with pain in my upper legs. They hurt a lot, and the pain is pretty constant. I'm an 85 year old male. Any suggestions? B from Independence

Dear B, in this case, it is virtually impossible for me to help much since I am unable to examine you, but let me offer some things to check.

First, assuming that there has been no trauma to the area where you're experiencing pain, you need to decide if this is joint pain, bone pain, or muscle pain. And, whether it is on one side or both sides.

If your pain is in your hip joint or joints, then the most common causes would be osteoarthritis or bursitis of the hips. Usually, these will cause tenderness when you press on the outside of the hip, pushing inward. If this is the case, then you might be able to get a joint injection from an orthopedic surgeon. Or, you can use over the counter maximum doses of acetaminophen and naproxen sodium. But, there is no cure for either osteoarthritis or bursitis. Unfortunately, that does not mean that the pain caused by these conditions is mild; far from it. The pain will wax and wane, but it can be a very intense, burning pain.

If the pain is one sided and feels like it is deep in the bone, then you need to go to your primary care provider and get an x-ray. There are conditions like avascular necrosis of the femoral head, or Paget's disease of the bone, or bone tumors like osteosarcoma. Happily, these are much less common, and they can be ruled out with a normal x-ray of the femur and/or hip.

Next, any time that we are considering muscle pain or weakness, we have to rule out medications that may be causing this. So, are you taking a statin? Examples are simvastatin (Zocor), atorvastatin (Lipitor), rosuvastatin (Crestor), etc. These drugs are wonderful if you have coronary artery disease, vascular disease, diabetes, or a history of strokes. Unfortunately, they can also cause muscle pain. So, if you are taking one of those or one of their "cousins" you probably need to stop or cut down the dose. Either way, you must discuss this with your doctor.

There are a few conditions that cause "proximal" muscle pain or more often muscle weakness. The word proximal means "near the center of the body," as opposed to "distal," which would be near the feet or the hands. Therefore, "proximal muscle" weakness or pain would be weakness/pain in the thighs, hip muscles, and/or the shoulder muscles. So, try to determine if your problem is pain or weakness and very importantly, try to determine if it is only in the thigh muscles or in other muscles.

If it is pain and is in your "proximal muscles" then there are three conditions that come to mind immediately. They are dermatomyositis, polymyositis and polymyalgia rheumatica. These conditions are "rheumatologic" and usually require the care of a rheumatologist. I believe that Dr. Karim Masri, who is a rheumatologist, has a "telemedicine clinic" at Wilson County Medical Center. (Of course, there are plenty of Rheumatologists in Tulsa, Wichita, or Kansas City.) Your primary care doctor may want to do some basic labs before sending you or they may just wait to have the rheumatologist do the testing. But, be thinking about whether you have had a new rash, or changes in your eye sight, and make sure that you pass that information on to the rheumatologist. There are other rheumatologic conditions like ankylosing spondylitis that is actually a disease of the sacroiliac joints, but it will cause hip girdle pain that can start in the low back and wrap around both sides, but again, a Rheumatologist is the person to see.

Of course, there are also multiple possible problems with your lumbar spine (like bulging discs, herniated discs, and degenerative vertebral disease in general) that can cause low back or hip pain that can also move down one thigh. It is rare that this would cause pain down both thighs, but it can happen. In that case, a Neurosurgeon is the one you need to see.

Unfortunately, sometimes we just can't find the cause of the pain. If that is the case, don't forget to try other treatments like chiropractic care, acupuncture, massage, and even hypnosis. Unless you have liver disease maximum dose acetaminophen (max dose is 3,000 mg/day) can really help. At the same time, and if you do not have kidney disease, congestive heart failure, or ulcers, you can take the maximum dose of either ibuprofen (max dose is 2,400 mg/day) OR the maximum dose of naproxen sodium (max dose is 1,500 mg/day). Max doses of acetaminophen with max dose NSAIDs can really keep your pain at a manageable level. I know that is not much, but I hope it helps.

Chapter 47

WHAT TO DO ABOUT AN EARWAX FACTORY

Dear Dr. Anne, In the midst of questions regarding cancer, stroke and heart attacks, this seems like an unimportant question, but apparently my ears are exceptionally productive earwax factories. Every couple of years I have to have the doctor clean them out. Is there anything that I can do to keep the earwax production under control? Signed B, from Independence.

Dear B, What a great question! And, it is an important question, because it is about quality of life. And, "YES!" there is something that you can do about earwax build up.

First, let me just say that our ears DO need to be cleaned out on a regular basis. It is actually NOT unusual for earwax to build up and get so bad that it reduces your hearing. For those who wear hearing aids, frequent ear cleaning is even more important, because the hearing aid seems to block the wax in and thus compound the buildup problem.

The important thing is to keep them clean WITHOUT sticking things deep down into your ear. So, I am NOT advocating sticking Q-Tips or anything else into your ear.

There are two approaches to treatment - dissolving the earwax or softening the earwax.

Dissolving the earwax can be accomplished with hydrogen peroxide. First, get a bottle of hydrogen peroxide, and a washcloth or some tissues. Lie down on your side, with your head on a pillow and pour about 1/3 of a capful of peroxide in your ear. Let it sit and bubble for about 3 to 5 minutes. Then hold the washcloth or tissues to the ear to catch the drainage and flip over. Repeat the process on the other ear. This costs almost nothing (a large bottle of hydrogen peroxide is about $1.50) and it is completely safe. You can do this as often as you like, even daily. If you really struggle with earwax production, I suggest you get in the habit of doing it often.

Another approach is to soften the earwax with mineral oil or glycerin. In this case, simply put a few drops in each ear before you go to sleep. You will want to have a towel over your pillow or you could end up with a bit of oil on your pillowcase. Again, these products are extremely inexpensive.

There are also over the counter products like Debrox. These products combine peroxide with an oil, and come with a dropper for easier dispensing. These also work great and I have prescribed them myself.

Some of us build up earwax "Shrek-style" and when you get it out you feel like you have enough to make a candle. Others deposit the wax in a large, flat "pancake" that can adhere to the skin. When these deposits are removed, they often pull a bit of skin with them and the ear will bleed. It is not a big deal, but it is very disconcerting for the patient.

When you have the doctor's office clean out your ear, they may use a Waterpik-like device that shoots a combination of warm water and hydrogen peroxide into the ear. It is usually not painful, but neither is it a comfortable process. If the Waterpik doesn't clear out the wax, they may use a little lighted tool to scrape the wax out, which is always uncomfortable. If those two efforts don't work, your primary care provider will likely send you to an Ear, Nose, and Throat specialist. Those guys have tools that the primary care doc's don't have.

The best option by far, is to avoid the whole problem by keeping your ears clean. Thanks for the question!

Chapter 48

WHAT ABOUT DAILY FIBER?

Dear Dr. Anne, my gastro-intestinal doctor tells me that I need to be taking fiber every day, but a lot of what I've read says it's best not to take extra fiber. Can you please clarify? Signed, W from Coffeyville.

Dear W, I see why you're puzzled. The "fiber question" is really confusing and even the "experts" very much disagree.

You've probably heard that old line about, "Fiber is a toothbrush for the colon – Keep your colon clean and get plenty of fiber every day!" Or maybe you haven't heard exactly that, but you surely have heard that a high fiber diet helps prevent colon cancer.

Well, you have heard that because in 1977, the United States Senate Select Committee on Nutrition and Human Needs laid out dietary goals of replacing animal products with grains as a way to "prevent cancer and heart disease." Most of us have grown up being told that we need huge amounts of fiber to keep our colons healthy.

Many gastroenterologists still recommend that their patients take fiber every day and I certainly consider them "experts" of the GI track. They usually recommend between 5 and 15 grams of fiber daily, or enough so that you never strain to have a BM. That is about 1 rounded teaspoon of Metamucil (or Konsyl, or something similar) between 1 and 3 times a day.

The problem is that there are a number of studies that have shown that fiber is actually not as beneficial as we have been told and in fact, may not be good at all. To start with, there was a study published in the *New England Journal of Medicine*, in January of 1999 that reported that fiber did nothing to improve "colon efficiency." Then *Lancet*, which is pretty much the ultimate technical journal on cancer, published an article in October of 2000, reporting that dietary fiber (even the ever popular soluble fiber) provided no protective benefit in preventing colon cancer.

This finding was "confirmed" in the "Wheat Bran Trial," published in 2002 by *Cancer Epidemiology, Biomarkers & Prevention*. That study randomly assigned patients to either a low fiber group (2 grams per day) or a high fiber group (13.5 grams per day). Here are some key findings from that study:

"No protective effect for adenoma recurrence was observed for those randomized to the high-fiber group as compared to those in the low-fiber group."

"Patients in the high-fiber intervention arm of the WBF (wheat bran fiber) trial reported side effects such as nausea, diarrhea, and abdominal bloating more frequently than those in the low fiber group."

"The results of this study show that neither fiber intake from a wheat bran supplement nor total fiber intake affects the recurrence of colorectal adenomas, thus lending further evidence to the body of literature indicating that consumption of a high-fiber diet, especially one rich in cereal fiber, does not reduce the risk of colorectal adenoma recurrence."

And there's one other very big concern. In 2000, The *Journal of Clinical Nutrition* reported that women eating the most fiber, along with the lowest amount of fat in their diet, have 20% lower calcium retention. "Natural sources of fiber, such as cereals and fruits, generally have a depressing effect on absorption of minerals such as calcium, iron, zinc, and copper."

So, the question in your mind may be, "Why are the GI doc's still pushing daily fiber supplementation?"

What I have found is that most are actually NOT prescribing fiber for everyone, across the board. They are prescribing fiber for those patients that have hemorrhoids, fissures, diverticulosis, or chronic constipation. For people who struggle with those issues, you need to take just enough fiber to keep you from having to strain when you poop.

We cannot digest cellulose like termites, nor can we ruminate like cows, and your colon doesn't really need a toothbrush. So, you don't need to push yourself to get more and more fiber. Just keep things moving reasonably.

Thanks for sending in the question, I hope that helps.

Chapter 49

RECOGNIZING HEART ATTACKS IN WOMEN

Dear Dr. Anne, a group of my girlfriends and I were talking the other day about our health and someone said something about heart attacks. We had all heard that women don't necessarily have the same symptoms as men, so how do we know when we are in trouble and need to go to the ER? Signed, E from Independence.

Dear E, you and your friends are completely right; men and women don't necessarily have the same symptoms when they are having a "heart attack." And, unfortunately, many women don't realize that cardiovascular disease is the leading cause of death in women. So, your question is a great one.

Let's start by clarifying some terms:

Infarction is the term used to describe the death of tissue due to inadequate blood supply to that particular area of tissue.

Myocardial infarction (MI), is the irreversible death of heart muscle due to prolonged lack of oxygen from insufficient blood supply. "Myo" means muscle. "Cardial" means of the heart. Infarction, again is tissue death because of inadequate blood supply. So, myocardial infarction is damage to the heart muscle.

Cardiovascular disease (CVD) and coronary artery disease (CAD) are essentially the same term. They both refer to the disease process that causes MI's. That is ruptured plaques in the arteries that supply blood to the heart muscle.

(By the way, heart failure is a completely different term and a different disease. Heart failure can be caused by an MI or repeated MI's. But let's save that topic for another day.)

The heart is a big muscle. When that muscle is not getting enough blood (and therefore, not enough oxygen) it is painful. Usually, people describe this as "crushing" chest pain. And, this chest pain is usually associated with exertion. If you are exerting yourself, then your heart is going to have to work harder and it will need more oxygen.

Your coronary arteries are the vessels that supply the heart muscle with blood. If you have plaque in one of those arteries and it ruptures, then it will likely clog the vessel and the blood supply to part of your heart will be cut off. Often, this feeling of crushing chest pain can be so bad that you feel like you can't get a breath. It often radiates up to the jaw, back or to the left arm. Sometimes that pain is so intense that you become, sweaty, and nauseated. These are the classic signs and symptoms of an MI. But, to be absolutely clear, here is the list quoted from a 2007 JAMA article:

"Typical" Chest Pain or Discomfort
1) Precordial chest discomfort, pain, heaviness, or fullness, possibly radiating to the arm, shoulder, back, neck, jaw, epigastrium, or other location;
2) Symptoms exacerbated by exertion or stress;
3) Symptoms may be relieved by rest or use of nitroglycerin; and
4) Symptoms associated with shortness of breath, diaphoresis (sweating), nausea or vomiting, and light-headedness.

But, as you mentioned, some people don't present in this way. Women can have those classic symptoms, but they may instead present with:

1) Middle or upper back pain, or jaw pain;
2) Shortness of breath;
3) Paroxysmal nocturnal dyspnea (this means that you get short of breath after you have been lying down for about 30 minutes)
4) Nausea and vomiting;
5) Indigestion and loss of appetite;
6) Weakness and fatigue;
7) Cough;
8) Dizziness; and
9) Palpitations

In addition, I am sure you have heard of "silent" MI's. These are heart attacks that cause no chest pain, but they are still a blockage that is causing death of myocardial muscle cells. These silent MI's are more typical in women or in patients who have diabetes. That is why, when a diabetic, or a woman comes to the hospital complaining of shortness of air, standard practice is to rule out an MI even if it turns out to be a lung problem, like a COPD (chronic obstructive lung disease) exacerbation. Think of it this way: diabetics get peripheral neuropathy, because the high blood sugars damage the nerves. Well, the high blood sugars are also causing damage to other nerves in the body, and those around the heart are no exception.

In summary, the National Heart, Lung, and Blood Institute (NHLBI) and the American Heart Association (AHA) in the "Act in Time to Heart Attack Signs" campaign, have listed the following as symptoms to prompt you to call 911:

1) Chest discomfort. Most myocardial infarctions involve discomfort in the center of the chest that lasts for more than a few minutes, or goes away and comes back. The

discomfort can feel like uncomfortable pressure, squeezing, fullness, or pain.

2) Discomfort in other areas of the upper body. Can include pain or discomfort in one or both arms, the back, neck, jaw, or stomach.

3) Shortness of breath. Often comes along with chest discomfort. But, it also can occur before chest discomfort.

4) Other symptoms. May include breaking out in a cold sweat, nausea, or light headedness.

The point is that if you are feeling a combination of those things described above, you need to go to the nearest emergency room and be checked out, on the double!

Chapter 50

HEART FAILURE PART 1

Dear Dr. Anne, In last week's column you said something about heart failure being completely different than heart attacks, but you didn't explain. I have always assumed that they are the same thing. Can you please explain the difference? Signed, F from Independence.

Dear F, I would love to! In case you never noticed, I love medicine. I love talking about it and writing about it. But, this may take a couple of columns, because there are several kinds of heart failure.

So, if we are going to understand heart failure, first we have to make sure that we know how the heart works. So, here are the basics. There are four chambers in the heart: the right and left atria, and the right and left ventricles labeled RA, LA, RV and LV, respectively in the picture below.

There are also 4 valves in the heart: the tricuspid valve is between the right atrium and the right ventricle. The pulmonary valve is between the right ventricle and the lungs. The mitral valve is between the left atrium and the left ventricle. And, finally, the aortic valve is between the left ventricle and the rest of the body.

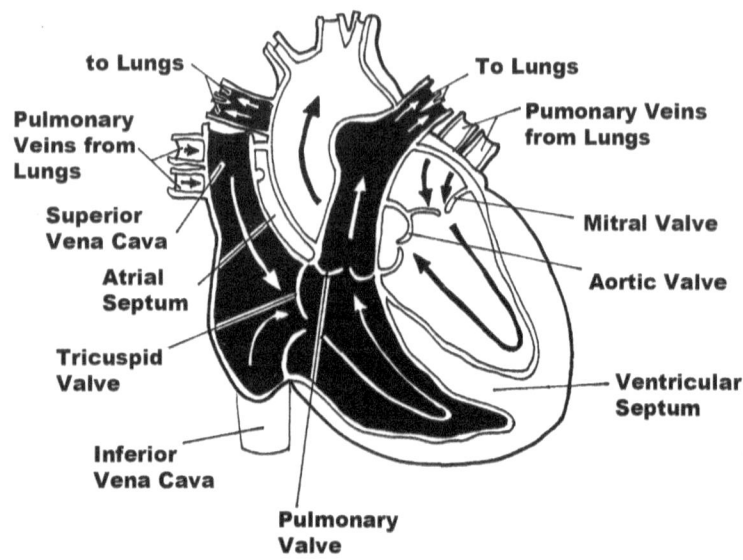

Blood enters the right atrium, through the superior vena cava and the inferior vena cava. It is pumped from the right atrium, into the right ventricle, and from there it is pumped into the lungs where it gives up its carbon dioxide and gets fresh oxygen. Coming back from the lungs, the blood enters the left atrium and is pumped into the left ventricle and from there, out to the whole body through the aortic valve and then the aorta.

Any time the heart is not able to supply enough blood to the body, we call it "heart failure." In general, the term heart failure refers to a *chronic* inability of the heart to supply the needs of the body. There are many reasons why this can happen. The classic cause of heart failure is when the muscle around the left ventricle becomes weak and is not strong enough to squeeze the blood out of the heart effectively. This can be caused by chronic heavy use of alcohol, by diabetes, or by scar tissue from previous myocardial infarctions. Alcohol and diabetes weaken the muscle. A previous MI causes the good muscle tissue to be replaced by scar tissue.

Last week we talked about the symptoms of myocardial infarctions (MI's). Again, an MI happens when there is a blockage in one of the vessels that supplies blood to the heart. In the drawing below, you can see that there is a "coronary occlusion," which just means that there is a blockage in one of the coronary arteries, or an artery that supplies the heart. The area below that will then "infarct," or die, because it is not getting enough blood.

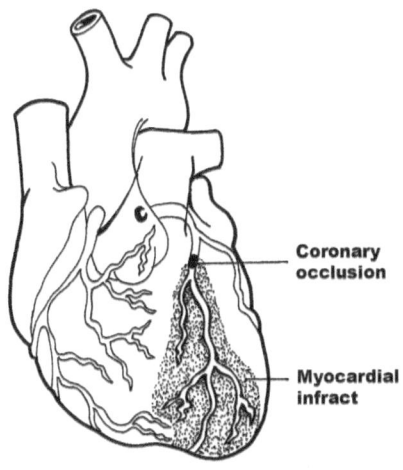

After a patient has an MI, the area that was infarcted will be rebuilt with scar tissue. Doctors call this remodeling. If you have a scar in the muscle of your thigh, it will be thin and fibrous and it will no longer contract like normal muscle. It is the same way with the heart. After an MI, the scarred area of the heart will not be able to contract and pump blood as well as the rest of the heart muscle. If the area is large, then the patient will end up with a large, but weak heart.

When someone comes to the ER reporting chest pain, this is why we work so hard to see if they are actually having an MI quickly. If we find evidence that they are, we rush them to the heart catheterization lab and stent the vessel open that has the blockage. Happily, we are doing a much better job of getting people to the heart cath lab quickly, so there is not as much heart muscle cell damage and cell death as there used to be. And, therefore, not as much resulting heart failure from previous MI's as there used to be.

In the picture below, you can see that the normal strong muscle of the left ventricle (shown in the first picture) has been replaced by thin scar tissue.

Systolic Failure

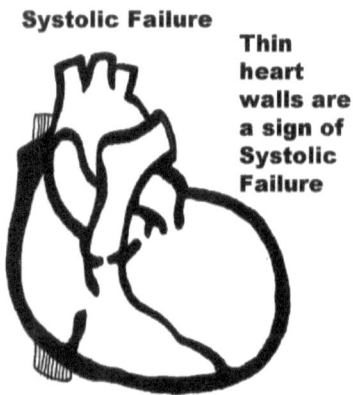

Thin heart walls are a sign of Systolic Failure

The thin scarred tissue of the remodeled left ventricle cannot squeeze properly. This causes "Systolic Heart Failure," which means that the left side of the heart is too weak to pump appropriately. (You could say that there is a failure in the squeezing ability of the heart.) Therefore, there is not going to be enough blood pumped out of the heart to supply the oxygen needs of the body, especially if the patient is exerting. So, the patient will experience shortness of air with exertion.

Moreover, think about the continuous loop of blood circulating through the heart and the body. If the muscle around the left ventricle is weak, then it will not be able to squeeze all the blood out of the left ventricle. When blood from the left atrium tries to enter the left ventricle, there will already be too much blood there, which will make the blood back up into the left atrium. Now, when the blood from the lungs tries to enter the left atrium, there will already be too much blood there, which will make the blood back up into the lungs. This is what happens when someone has a "heart failure exacerbation." That means that we have to give them medications to force their kidneys to make more urine so that we reduce the blood volume and therefore, reduce the back up of blood in the lungs.

In summary, systolic heart failure is one type of heart failure. And, a big MI, multiple small MIs, chronic alcohol use, and diabetes can all lead to future systolic or left sided heart failure.

Chapter 51

HEART FAILURE PART 2

Last week we covered Systolic Heart Failure. To review, systolic heart failure happens when the left ventricle is too weak to effectively pump the blood throughout the body. I probably should have said this last week, but the "systolic" phase of the pumping of the heart is the squeezing phase. So, when the left ventricle is weak it can't squeeze well. In that case, the body tissues are not getting optimal blood supply, and this condition is called "Systolic Heart Failure."

I am repeating the drawing below to refresh your memory on the different chambers and valves of the heart and how the blood moves through the heart.

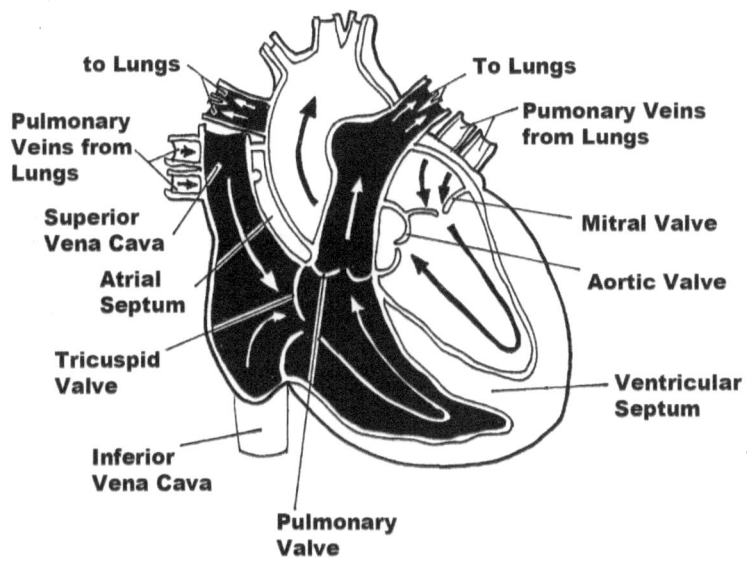

to Lungs

Pulmonary
Veins from
Lungs

Superior
Vena Cava

Atrial
Septum

Tricuspid
Valve

Inferior
Vena Cava

Pulmonary
Valve

To Lungs

Pumonary Veins
from Lungs

Mitral Valve

Aortic Valve

Ventricular
Septum

Today, I am going to explain the second major kind of heart failure, which is "Diastolic Heart Failure." The diastolic phase of the pumping of the heart is the relaxing phase. The right and left ventricles have to relax to accept the blood.

Think about filling a balloon with air. If the balloon is a round or oval shape the sides expand easily as you blow in the air. But, if the balloon is one of those long skinny ones, then the sides of the balloon don't relax and the only way to fill the balloon is when the air moves down into the "hot dog" shape.

So, if a person has had untreated or inadequately treated high blood pressure for many years, then the heart muscle has been working extra hard to push the blood out against high pressure. As a result, the muscle surrounding the left ventricle is now big and thick and stiff. You might think that a big, thick heart muscle is good, but it's not. Big muscles are only great when they are men's pec's and biceps. In the heart, a big thick muscle is not good, because it is stiff and cannot relax and accept enough blood. Think of the balloon again. Picture trying to blow up one of those skinny balloons, but now it has the same length as the round balloons. So, the sides of the balloon just won't relax enough for you to blow in much air.

Even if the heart is strong and has the ability to squeeze really hard, if the amount of blood coming in with each cycle is only half of what it should be, then it is still only going to pump out half of what it should. This means that there still isn't enough blood being pumped out to adequately supply the needs of the body.

The picture on the right is a repeat of last week showing "Systolic Heart Failure," when the muscle surrounding the left ventricle is weak and thin and floppy, because is it fibrous with scar tissue and has very little muscle left. I repeated this picture so that you could compare these two kinds of heart failure. The drawing on the left shows "Diastolic Heart Failure" where the muscle surrounding the left ventricle has gotten too thick and stiff, which is also called hypertrophy.

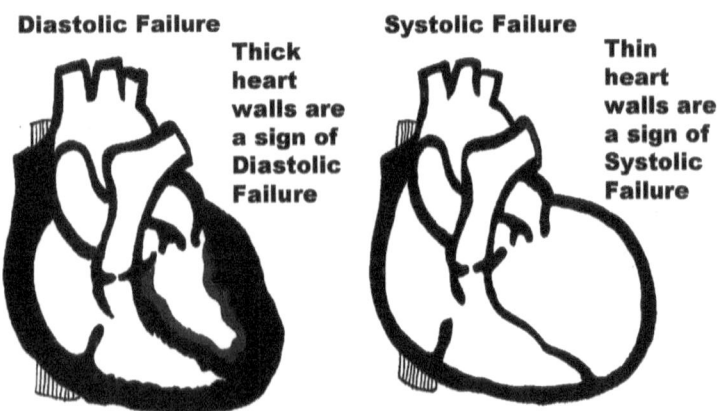

I need to stop here for the today, but next week we will finish diastolic heart failure. Again, diastolic heart failure means that the cardiac output is too low, because the heart is not able to relax and accept enough blood to adequately supply the needs of the body even though it is squeezing well.

Chapter 52

HEART FAILURE PART 3

Ok, we are almost finished with heart failure. You can see why I hadn't tackled heart failure before, right? It's complicated, but pretty darn interesting, isn't it?

Anyway, we need to talk more about diastolic heart failure. To review, the diastolic phase of the heart is the relaxation phase. So, when there is diastolic heart failure, the heart muscle is too thick and stiff to relax and accept enough blood. No matter how strongly the heart can squeeze, the cardiac output will still be low because there is not enough blood in the ventricle to begin with. Here I am repeating the anatomy of the heart if you need to review.

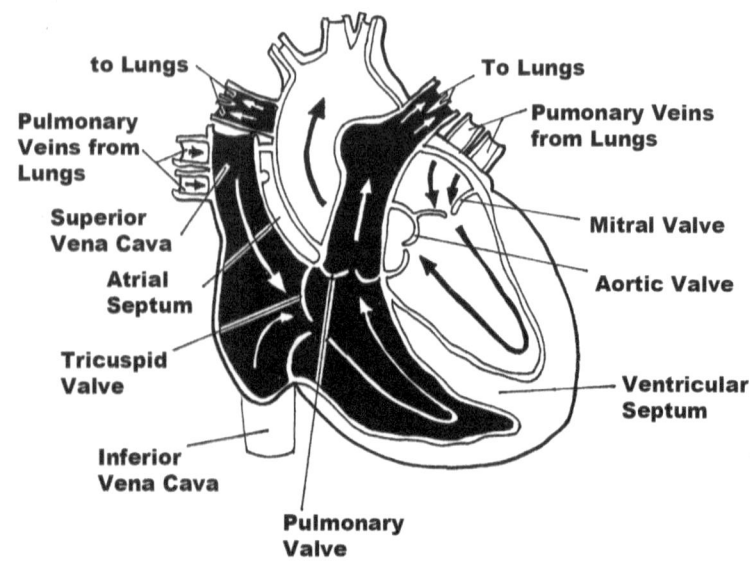

Diastolic heart failure is becoming increasingly common. As I said last week, it is often caused by long standing poorly treated high blood pressure. But, it can also be caused by valvular disease.

Review the picture above from the last two columns, and notice the aortic valve. You can see that the blood leaving the left ventricle has to go through the aortic valve. As we age, the body will often deposit calcium on this valve. The calcium makes the valve incredibly stiff and hard to open. If this happens, you can see how the muscle surrounding the left ventricle will end up being big and thick because it has to constantly push against the ever hardening aortic valve. The picture below is actually more accurate than the one last week. Do you see how small the left ventricle is?

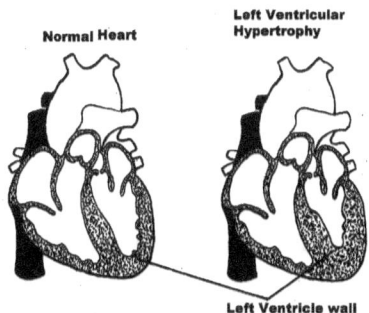

Now, think about the blood coming back from the lungs and trying to enter the left atrium. If the left ventricle is small because the muscle has hypertrophied, then not all of the blood from the atrium will fit in the ventricle. This means that the blood coming into the left atrium is going to hit a traffic jam. There is no place for it to go. This means that blood coming from the lungs will also have no place to go, which means the blood is going to start backing up in the lungs and the patient will be increasingly short of breath.

Now think about another scenario. What if you used to smoke cigarettes? (I know you have quit or are at least cutting way back, right?) Say that you quit when you turned 55, but you started when you were about 20 years old. That means that your lungs have been damaged. You may not need supplemental oxygen or inhalers, but your lungs are undoubtedly stiff. That means the muscle surrounding the right ventricle has had to push really hard to get the blood from the right ventricle into the lungs. Check out the picture below.

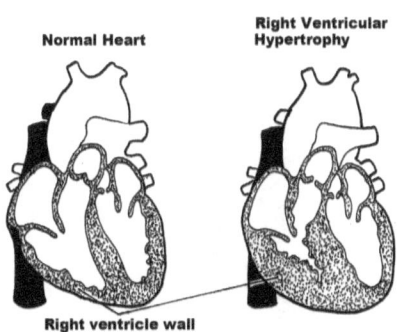

Look how tiny the right ventricle is. Go back up to the first picture and find the right atrium and recall that the blood from the whole body enters the heart at the right atrium. From the right atrium, the blood is pumped down to the right ventricle. But, if the right ventricle is so tiny, then all the blood from the right atrium won't fit in it. When that happens, the blood obviously backs up in the right atrium. So, when more blood tries to enter the right atrium, there is no room. So, what is going to happen? The blood will back up into the legs.

So, heart failure can cause fluid to back up in the lungs and in the legs. The symptoms will be fatigue, shortness of air, and swelling (also called edema) and in this case it will become pitting edema.

Congestive Heart Failure

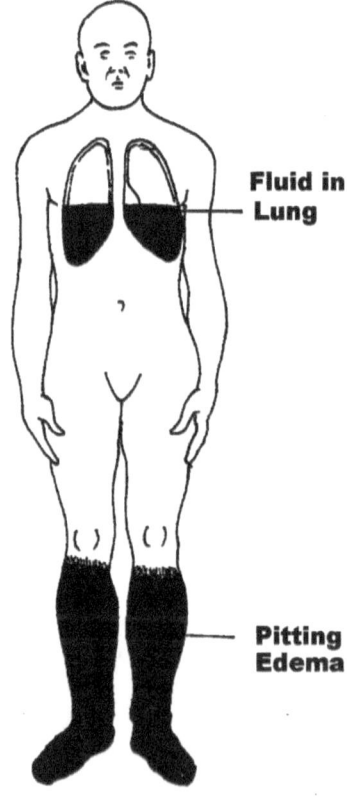

Fluid in Lung

Pitting Edema

Heart failure is not easy to manage; there is a lot to it. Of course, if you can avoid getting there in the first place, you are much better off. If you already have some form of heart failure, there is a class about living with heart failure that is offered periodically at CRMC and it is really worthwhile.

The most important thing is to control your blood pressure if you have hypertension, and stop smoking if you are a smoker. If you can't completely quit, then cut down on the number of cigarettes whenever possible. Exercise daily; you don't need to run a marathon, just do what you can. I don't care if all you do is walk around the couch during commercials. Start there, and increase by baby steps. And if your feet and legs start to swell, wear compression socks.

There are still other things to say about heart failure, but these are the big ones. I hope this helps.

Chapter 53

WHAT'S UP WITH SKIN TAGS?

Dear Dr. Anne, what's the deal with skin tags? I don't want them! Signed, D from Independence.

Dear D from Independence, Thanks for writing in. Skin tags are just weird aren't they? Here's a picture showing a skin tag for anyone who is not sure what they look like.

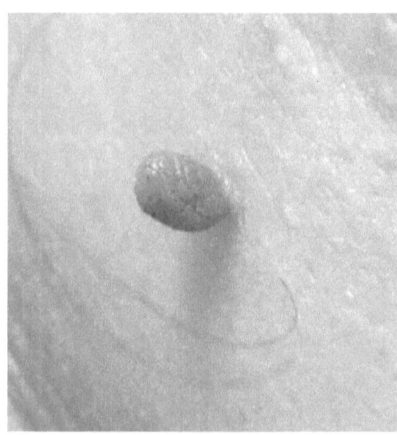

Skin tags are also called acrochordons. Most importantly, they are benign, that means they are NOT cancerous. They are very common (about 50% of adults get them) and they usually happen in areas where the skin gets rubbed. For example, under the arm,

or on the neck, or in the groin, etc. It is interesting that they can increase during the second trimester of pregnancy, but will usually disappear after the baby is born. They also seem to frequently be related to insulin resistance in type II diabetes.

Skin tags can turn dark, if they get twisted and the blood supply is cut off. This is not a huge deal, the tag will die and fall off. Just make sure it doesn't get infected, so have your doc check it.

Skin tags can be easily removed by several methods, clipping them off, cauterizing, etc. I would love to tell you that it is fine to yank these little guys off yourself, but they should be distinguished from two other very similar looking lesions. The first is called a pedunculated dermal nevus (which is a kind of mole) and the second is a neurofibroma (which is small skin tumor). So, if you notice something that you think might be a skin tag, have your doctor look it over. Unfortunately, insurance may not pay for the removal of skin tags since they are benign.

And, by the way, if I haven't gotten to your question, don't give up on me. I have a list that I am slowly plowing through. However, if it has been a while, there is always a chance that I have lost it, so feel free to remind me. Until then, thanks for your questions. I love medicine and I hope you do to!